# Latest Developments in Medical Robotics Systems

*Edited by Serdar Küçük*

Published in London, United Kingdom

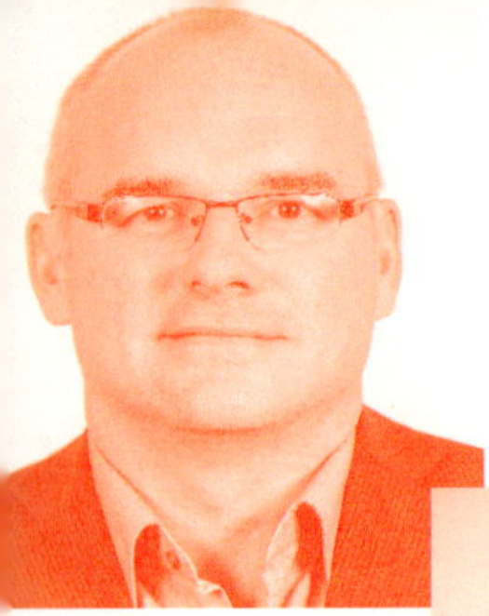
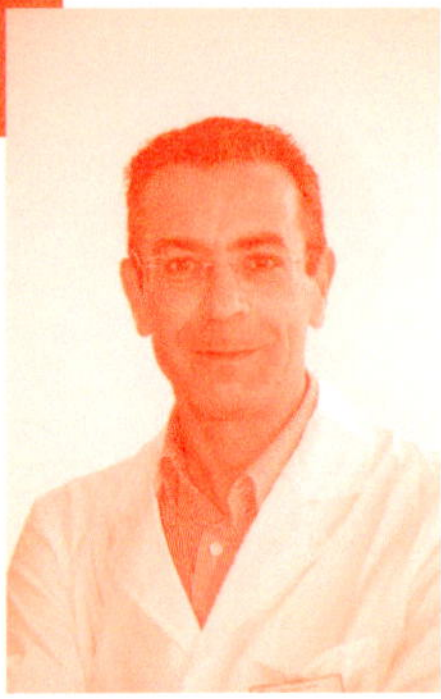
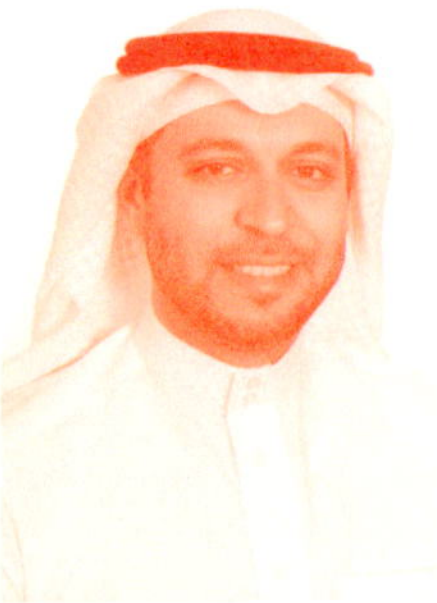
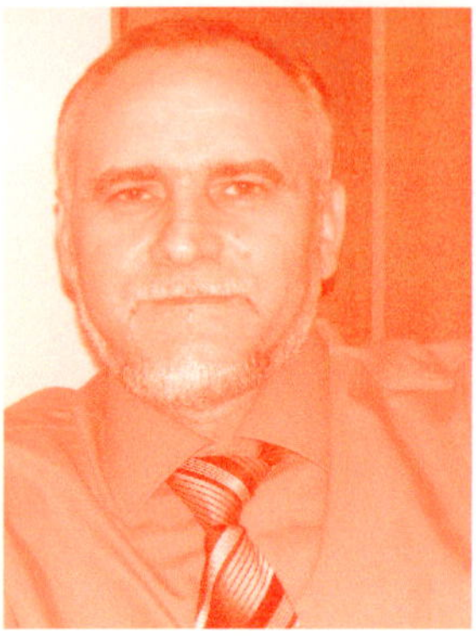
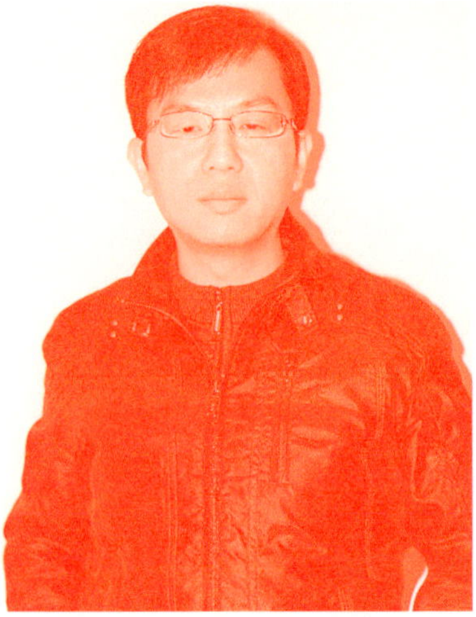
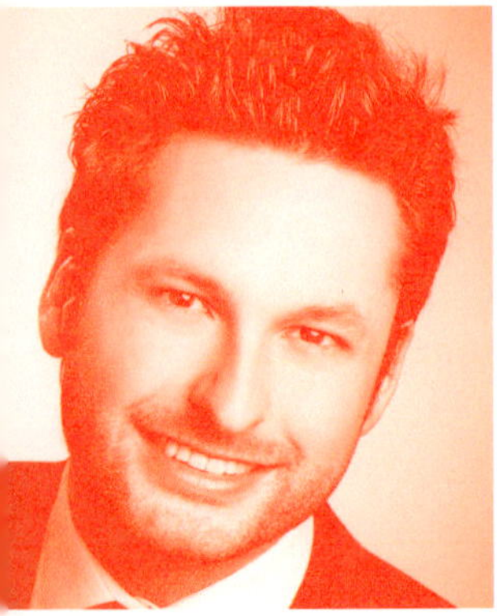
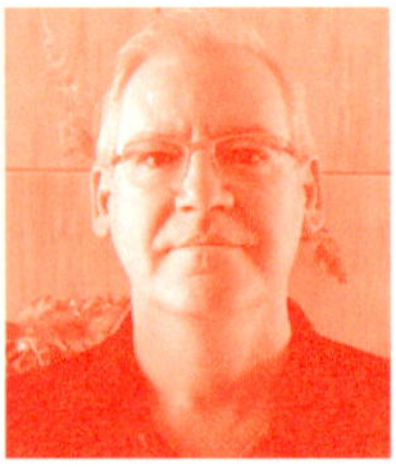

IntechOpen

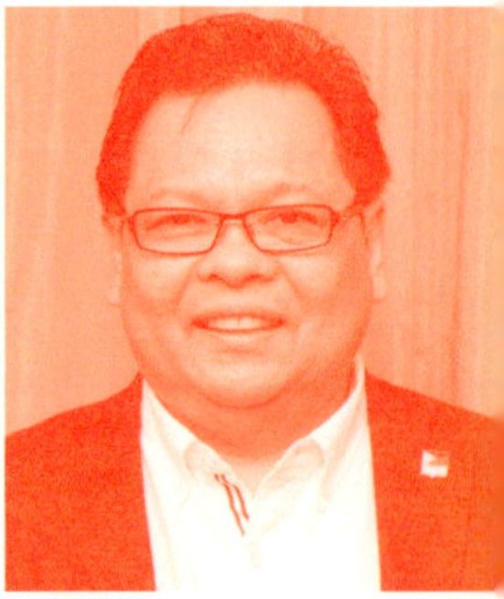
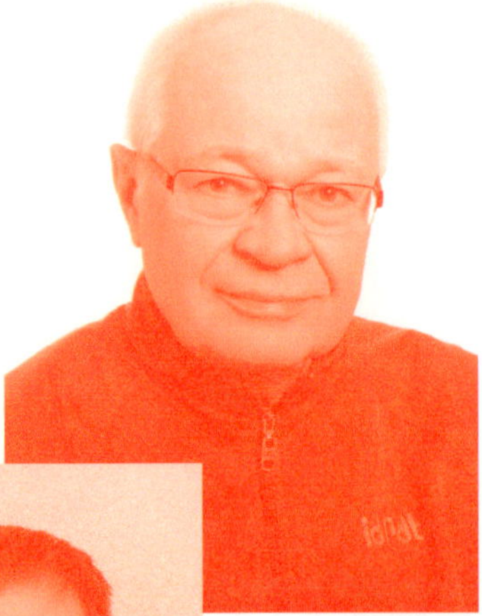
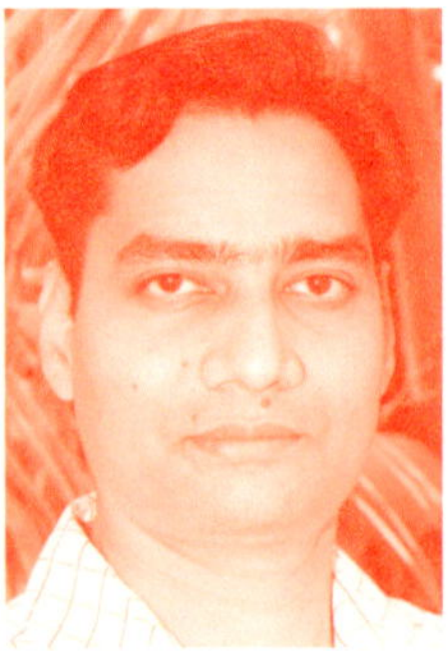
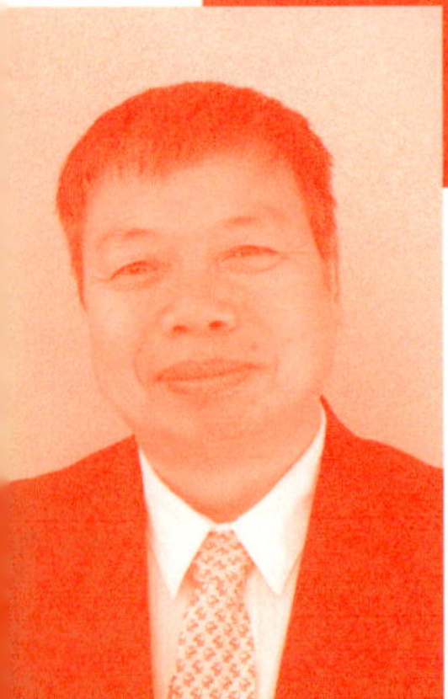
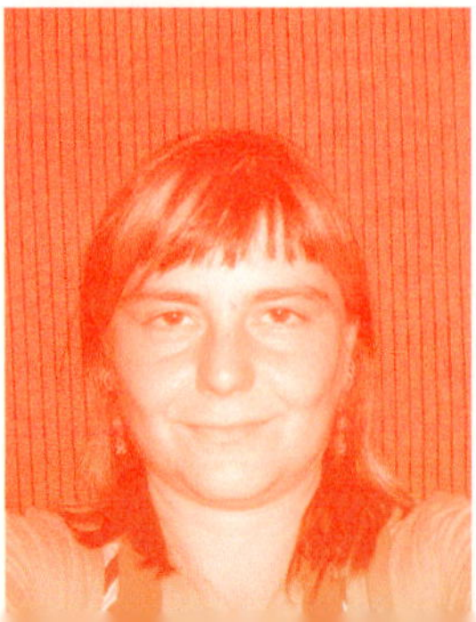
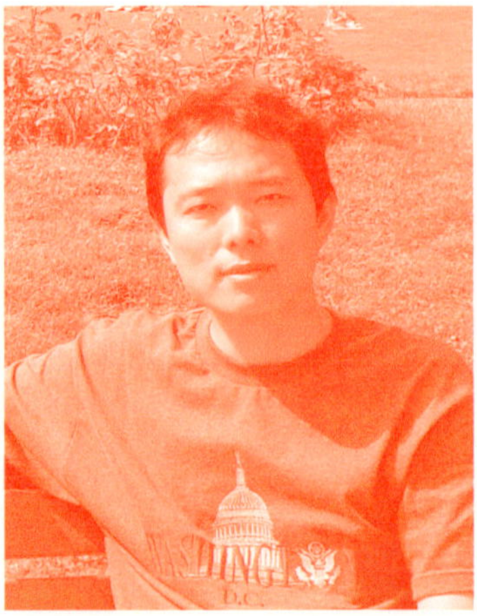

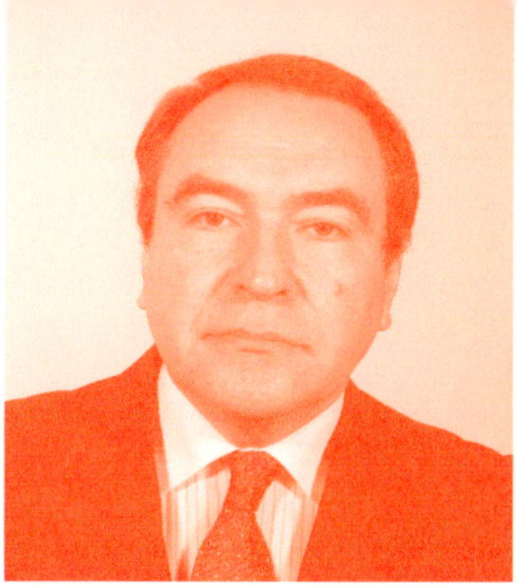
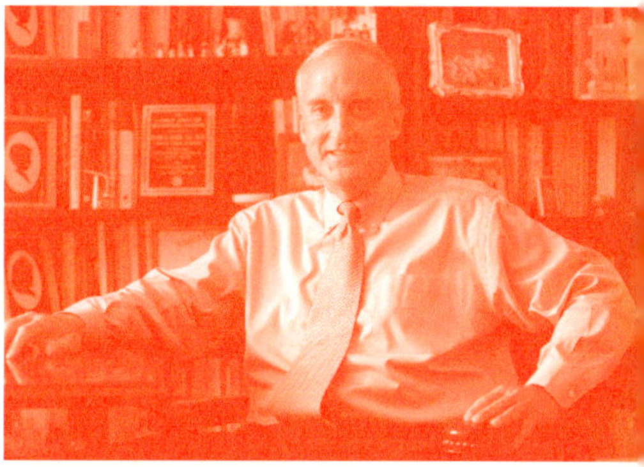
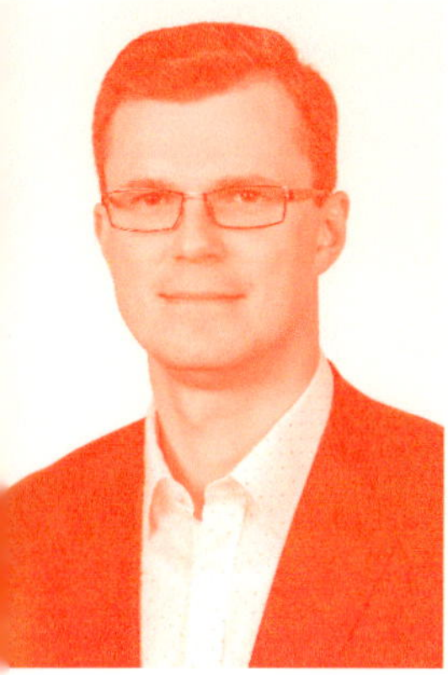
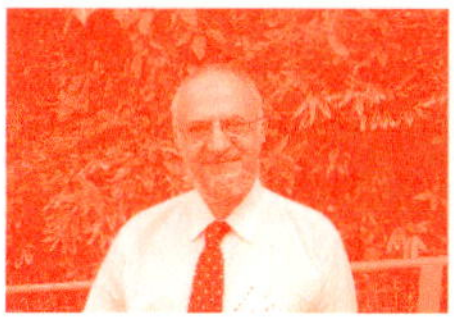
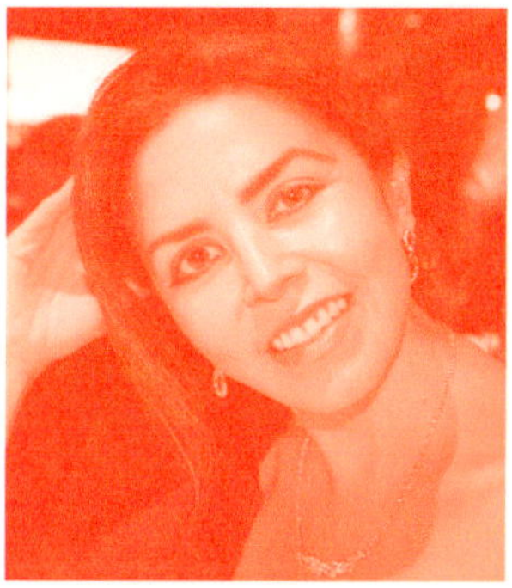

*Supporting open minds since 2005*

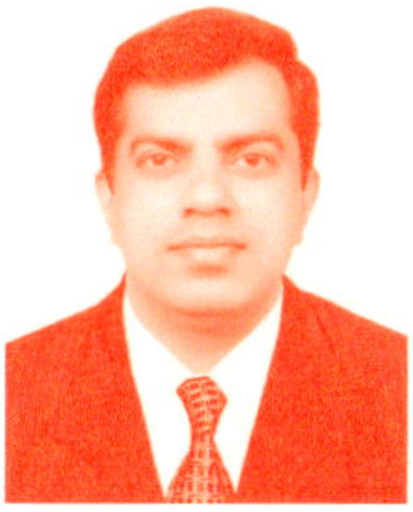
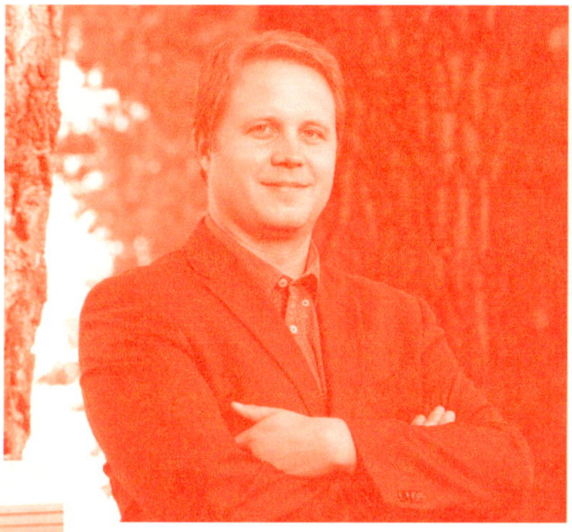
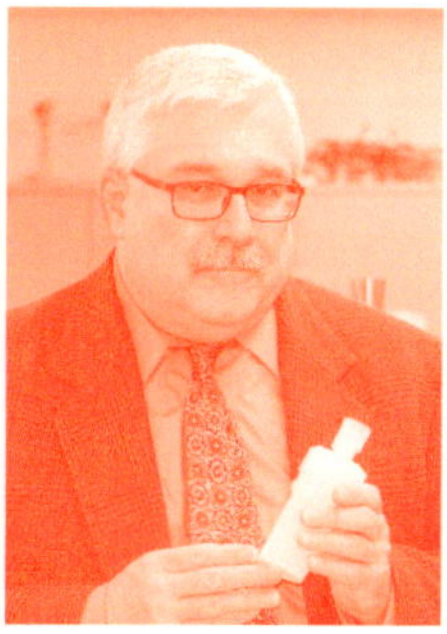
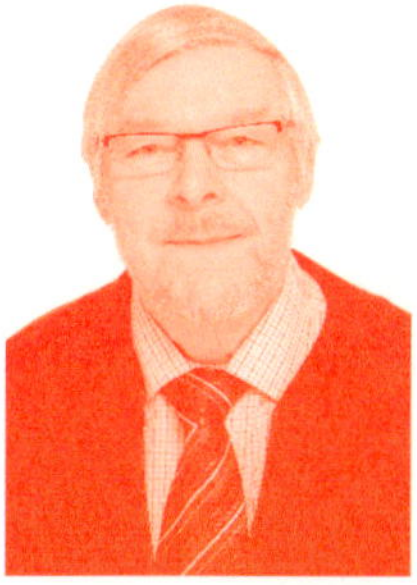
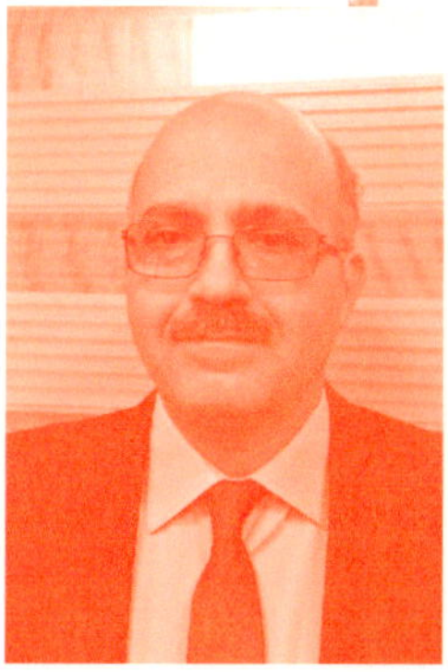
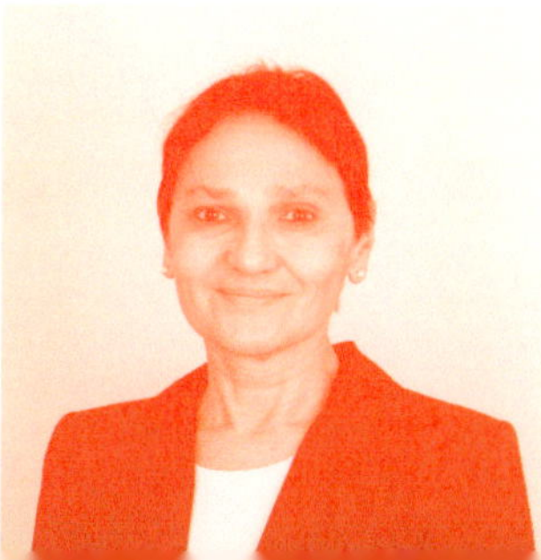
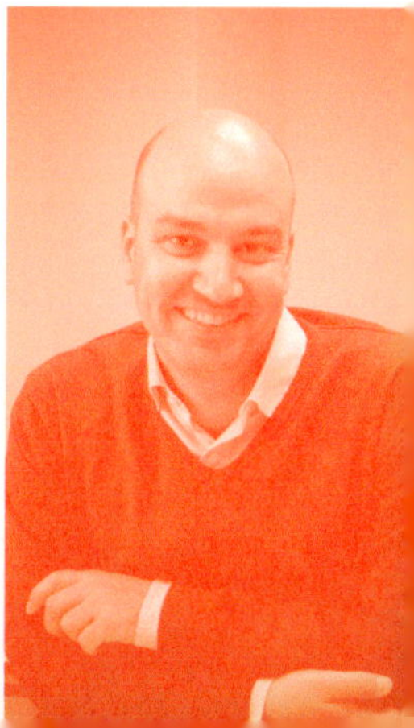

Latest Developments in Medical Robotics Systems
http://dx.doi.org/10.5772/intechopen.92945
Edited by Serdar Küçük

Contributors
Ekin Guran, Gianluca Torregrossa, Andrea Amabile, Mario Navarrete-Arellano, Radamés Rivas López, Rafael Diaz-Nieto, Mushfique Alam, Robert Young, Tony Boiadjiev, George Boiadjiev, Kamen Delchev, Ivan Chavdarov, Rumen Kastelov, Jeroen M.H. Hendriks, Lawek Berzenji, Krishan Yogeswaran, Patrick Lauwers, Paul Van Schil, Alan Lumsden, Marton Berczeli, Peter Legeza, Pranjal Desai, Ryan Gillentine, Serdar Küçük



First published in London, United Kingdom, 2021 by IntechOpen
IntechOpen is the global imprint of INTECHOPEN LIMITED, registered in England and Wales, registration number: 11086078, 5 Princes Gate Court, London, SW7 2QJ, United Kingdom
Printed in Croatia

British Library Cataloguing-in-Publication Data
A catalogue record for this book is available from the British Library

Additional hard and PDF copies can be obtained from orders@intechopen.com

Latest Developments in Medical Robotics Systems
Edited by Serdar Küçük
p. cm.
Print ISBN 978-1-83969-382-3
Online ISBN 978-1-83969-383-0
eBook (PDF) ISBN 978-1-83969-384-7

For EU product safety concerns:
IN TECH d.o.o., Prolaz Marije Krucifikse Kozulić 3, 51000 Rijeka, Croatia, info@intechopen.com or visit our website at intechopen.com.

# Meet the editor

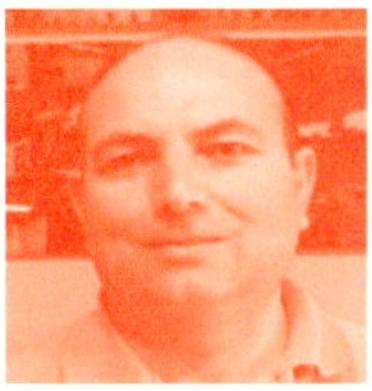

Serdar Küçük received a BA and MSc from Marmara University, Istanbul, Turkey, in 1995 and 1998, respectively. He received a Ph.D. from Kocaeli University, Turkey, in 2004, where he is currently a full professor in the Department of Biomedical Engineering. He has several scientific publications to his credit, including international conference papers, journal papers, books, and book chapters. He serves as a reviewer for several well-known robotic journals. He is also an editor of scientific books. His research interests include optimization, control, and kinematics and dynamics modelling of serial and parallel robotic manipulators. Lately, Dr. Kucuk has also been interested in designing electrically controlled, above-knee prosthetics and hand–wrist rehabilitation robots, surgical robots, and biomedical robotic devices.

# Contents

# Preface

Medical robots have significant potential for treating patients quickly and comfortably. Medical professionals increasingly prefer robotic technology because of its utility for several medical applications. Medical robots are employed for surgical operations, such as cardiac surgery, prostate surgery, plastic surgery, kidney surgery, and more. They are especially preferred for surgery over traditional methods because they present better results, including smaller incisions, greater accuracy, and shortened recovery time. Medical robots are also used for several other procedures such as transporting blood from one place to another, preparing substances in a hazardous environment, diagnosing illnesses, and caring for patients.

Robotic technology is at a very interesting point, especially in terms of medical robots. The replacement of medical personnel by robots may be inevitable. Every passing year, many new robotic designs are developed to help people of all ages, from children to the elderly. This book presents the latest developments in medical robotics and innovative designs of the future. It also examines current medical robotic systems and applications.

I would like to thank all authors who contributed to this book with their valuable novel ideas and their knowledge of current developments in medical robotics.

**Serdar Küçük, Ph.D.**
Full Professor,
Technology Faculty,
Department of Biomedical Engineering,
Kocaeli University,
Turkey

Section 1

# Introduction

Chapter 1

# Introductory Chapter: Future of Medical Robots

*Serdar Küçük*

## 1. Introduction

In real life, most of us perform repetitive tasks in factories, school, hospitals and so on. Several people do not like these kinds of tasks and get bored from working offices as well as their jobs. Especially, medical staffs in the hospitals perform thousands of repetitive tasks such as draw blood, make dental filling, visualize patients' vital signs like measuring the human heart rate. Medical staffs make never-ending diagnosis, prevention, and treatment of diseases. As the average life expectancy increases day by day in the world, people are getting older. As the people getting older, the number of patients is increasing more than in the past. As a result of this increase, surgeons execute never-ending surgeries under the pressure of performance; laboratory workers perform never-ending urine and blood tests and dentists always tirelessly remove build-up or decay from teeth. It is possible to multiply these examples.

Being in a hospital is a very stressful experience even in the best occasion. Especially waiting the medical treatment on the que is a tiring practice. In addition, being treated on time is directly related to the country's health staff and technical opportunities. In most countries in the world, due to the lack of medical staff or technique equipment, even for a simple dental filling, sometimes it is necessary to wait in line for months. Medical personnel are often physically and mentally fed up with this endless intensity. At this very moment, medical robots come to the aid of both patients and healthcare professionals.

As an example, robotic medical staffs like robotic nurses, robotic laboratory devices, robotic surgeons can fulfill the boring tasks mention above. Robots are the best candidates to execute the repetitive, monotonous and dangerous tasks without being bored, tired and overwhelmed. According to the market investigations, the market size of surgical robots alone has already exceeded 5 billion dollars.

## 2. Medical robots transforming the healthcare system

Almost 80 years have passed since the development of the first robot manipulator. Robots, which were originally produced only for industrial purposes, have spread to many areas over time. Today, robots have become equipped enough to work alone in a factory, skilled enough to participate in operations in a hospital, and smart enough to bring a selected product from a shopping mall. The rise of robotic technology and the replacement of workers by robots has become an inevitable reality. It has now become impossible to prevent the development of robotic technology. Now, robots have gained the competence to work in the same office with humans. In the near future, it seems inevitable that some people will completely leave their jobs to robots [1, 2]. At this


IntechOpen

point, the following question comes to mind. How ready is humanity for this inevitable future? What kind of solutions do social scientists propose for this inevitable future in the world?

The fact that robots have become such advanced devices has had very beneficial results for humanity. Some of these are better diagnosis for everyone, safer surgery, more advanced and yet cheaper prosthetic legs, shorter waiting times and lower infection rates. Some main areas where robots will be employed, especially in the health sector, can be listed as follows: Robot assisted surgery, medical micro robots, rehabilitation robots, advanced protheses and robotic nurses.

### 2.1 Robot assisted surgery

Until recently, surgeons were performing operations using traditional methods. The most important disadvantage of these traditional methods was to perform the operations by making very large incisions in the patient's body. Therefore, the traditional method has many disadvantages, from esthetic appearance to late recovery. Robot-assisted surgery can eliminate these disadvantages. Robot-assisted surgery is performed as follows: Small incisions are made on the patient's body for the surgeon to operate on the patient using a robot. Surgical instruments and camera are placed to the body from these small cuts. The surgeon performs the surgery using these surgical instruments from a remote console. Since the operated area is magnified several times by means of the camera, the surgeon has the opportunity to see the operational region in more detail than the traditional methods. Thus, the surgeon performs a more comfortable and successful operation. Minimally invasive surgery using robots provides many advantages over traditional methods: i) patient recovers in a shorter time, ii) the surgeon sees the operated area in higher resolution, iii) patients have less risk of infections, iv) the patient returns to his/her traditional life more quickly, and v) economic cost is reduced because the patient is treated in a shorter time. The most famous robotic system used in minimally invasive surgery is definitely the Vinci Surgical System which is used several operations like in cardiac surgery, general surgery, gynaecologic surgery, thoracic surgery, and urologic surgery [3].

### 2.2 Medical micro robots

Treatment with medical microrobots is an area that medicine has just encountered. These new robotic devices, which are not very similar to the structure of traditional industrial robots, are used to solve the problem in a certain region in patient's body. In general, medical micro robots with spiral tails reach the sick area in the human body by moving through blood vessels. Using this method, the drug can be applied only to the affected area. Thus, healthy area can be prevented from the drug.

### 2.3 Rehabilitation robots

Rehabilitation robots are intelligent machines designed to help patients regain their lost skills. Rehabilitation robots are used to restore the lost sensorimotor functions, especially in the arms, hands and legs, by making the patient perform programmed exercises. Robotic rehabilitation devices, which are getting more functional every passing day, are used to restore lost skills in the lower and upper extremities. Currently, many types of rehabilitation robots are produced for the rehabilitation of lower and upper extremity regions. Some important commercially produced lower extremity rehabilitation robotic systems can be listed as Lokohelp [4] and Lokomat [5]. On the other hand, some upper extremity rehabilitation robotic systems can be listed as Esa human arm exoskeleton [6], L-exos [7] and Sarcos Master Arm [8].

### 2.4 Advanced prostheses

Traditional prostheses are devices that allow amputees to perform basic movements while walking. Therefore, traditional prostheses cannot fully perform human hand, arm and wrist movements. More complex and advanced systems are needed to fully imitate the movements of a healthy person with a prosthesis. Prosthetics with sensors and actuators are good candidate robotic mechanisms to fully mimic human movements. Humanity has come to a point where more performance can be achieved than natural limbs with new generation robotic prostheses. Humanity is at a point where it can perform the act of feeling apart from actions such as walking, holding and lifting with prostheses [9–12].

### 2.5 Robotic nurses

Nurses are the worker bees of the healthcare system. It is almost inevitable to encounter at least one nurse next to the doctors in every hospital room where diagnosis and treatment is made. With the increase in life expectancy, older people inevitably spend their last days in hospital rooms or nursing homes. As a result, aging creates an increasing workload for nurses. It seems that robot nurses will come to the rescue of nurses who are overwhelmed by this workload. Robotic nurses can monitor and record vital signs, monitor the patient's condition and report the situation to the responsible health personnel. Robotic nurses are not only candidates to be the best friends of the elderly people, but also seem to be candidates for jobs of human nurses.

## 3. Conclusions

As a result of the rapid digitalization of the world, robots are also becoming more capable at an increasing rate. As the designs of medical robots are becoming more useful day by day, there is a significant decrease in costs compared to the past. As a result of the decrease in robot costs, robots are turning into candidates for the jobs of healthcare professionals. Although robots are increasingly taking their place in the healthcare system, the social consequences of this are not yet fully understood. If healthcare personnel will work less in the future, how healthcare personnel will spend their free time is a phenomenon that social scientists should consider in advance.

## Author details

Serdar Küçük
Department of Biomedical Engineering, Technology Faculty, Kocaeli University, Turkey

*Address all correspondence to: skucuk@kocaeli.edu.tr

## References

[1] Küçük, Ö.- Industry 4.0, Artificial Intelligence and New Period of Labour Relations, 10th International Symposium on Intelligent Manufacturing and Service System, 60-68, 2019.

[2] Küçük, Ö.- Artificial intelligence, fierce competition and crime prevention policy in post -industrial labor relations, International Crimes and History, Issue: 20, 121-161, 2019.

[3] Dwivedi J, Mahgoub I. Robotic surgery - A review on recent advances in surgical robotic systems, Florida Conference on Recent Advances in Robotics, 2012. Boca Raton, Florida, May 10-11, 2012.

[4] Freivogel S, Mehrholz J, Husak-Sotomayor T, Schmalohr D. Gait training with the newly developed "LokoHelp"-system is feasible for non-ambulatory patients after stroke, spinal cord and brain injury. A feasibility study. Brain Injury. 2008;22(7-8):625-632

[5] Colombo G, Joerg M, Schreier R, Dietz V. Treadmill training of paraplegic patients using a robotic orthosis. Journal of Rehabilitation Research and Development. 2000;37(6):693-700

[6] Schiele A, Visentin G. The ESA human arm exoskeleton for space robotics telepresence. In: Conference: International Symposium on Artificial Intelligence, Robotics and Automation in Space (iSAIRAS); Nara, Japan. Vol. 7. 2003

[7] Frisoli A, Bergamasco M, Carboncini C, Carboncini C, Rossi B. Robotic assisted rehabilitation in virtual reality with the L-EXOS. Studies in Health Technology and Informatics. 2009;145:40-54

[8] Michael Mistry, Peyman Mohajerian, Stefan Schaal, An Exoskeleton Robot for Human Arm Movement Study, 2005 IEEE/RSJ International Conference on Intelligent Robots and Systems (IROS 2005). 2005

[9] Ege, M., & Kucuk, S. Design and dynamic model of a novel powered above knee prosthesis. In 2019 Medical technologies congress (TIPTEKNO) (pp. 1-4). IEEE. October 2019.

[10] Ege, M., Küçük, S., & Memişoğlu, K. Trajectory planning of electronically controlled prosthesis by using third-order polynomial. In 2017 Medical technologies National Congress (TIPTEKNO) (pp. 1-4). IEEE. October 2017.

[11] Lee, J. T., Bartlett, H. L., & Goldfarb, M. Design of a semipowered stance-control swing-assist transfemoral prosthesis. IEEE/ASME Transactions on Mechatronics, 25(1), 175-184. 2019.

[12] Lenzi, T., Cempini, M., Hargrove, L. J., & Kuiken, T. A. Design, development, and validation of a lightweight nonbackdrivable robotic ankle prosthesis. IEEE/ASME Transactions on Mechatronics, 24(2), 471-482. 2019.

Section 2

# Robotic Assisted Surgery A

Chapter 2

# Robotic Liver Surgery

*Mushfique Alam, Robert Young and Rafael Diaz-Nieto*


## Abstract

Minimally invasive surgery has experienced a significant expansion in the last decades. Robotic surgery has evolved in parallel to traditional laparoscopic surgery offering additional technical advantages. Some specific aspect of Hepatobiliary Surgery led to a limited implementation of minimally invasive liver surgery in the early years of laparoscopic surgery whilst we are experiencing an exponential increase in the use of minimally invasive approaches to this type of intervention. In this chapter we describe the key aspect of robotic liver surgery with a meticulous description of the supporting evidence, its limitation and future perspectives.


**Keywords:** robotic surgery, robotic liver resection, hepatectomy, minimally invasive surgery, laparoscopic liver surgery

## 1. Introduction

Hepatic resection is the gold standard treatment for some of the most common malignant tumours of the liver, including primary tumours (hepatocellular carcinoma and cholangiocarcinoma) and colorectal liver metastasis and it can be sometimes the treatment option for some benign tumours [1]. Hepatobiliary surgery also includes complex biliary interventions for benign and malignant pathologies that, in addition to the liver resection, may require biliary reconstructions and bilioenteric anastomosis [2].

Open surgery remains the predominant approach for most of these hepatobiliary procedures. However, there is an exponential increase of minimally invasive surgery (MIS) within this field, supported by large cases series and randomised control trials (RCTs) recently published in the literature [3].

Outcomes from the available literature suggests that MIS for liver resections improves patients' outcomes in terms of length of stay, blood loss and postoperative complications. Although some series suggest longer operative time and higher initial costs, the overall cost-efficiency seems to favour laparoscopic surgery [4, 5]. Despite this data, laparoscopic liver surgery is not routinely performed in all Hepatobiliary Centres and there is a large proportion of patients being treated via open approach. The delayed implementation of this type of intervention is commonly related to the technical challenges of these operations, the long tradition of open surgery associated to liver transplantation and the specific technological requirements attached to this type of resections.

From the original era of the pioneers in laparoscopic surgery, the consensus meetings in Louisville and Morikawa highlighted the challenges of this new approach. Recommendations from these meetings were very cautious about suggesting laparoscopic liver surgery for every patient and limited its clear indication to minor resections. From them, MIS for minor liver resections (less than 3 segments) such as left lateral secitonectomy and segmentectomies from the anterior Couinaud segments (II to VI) became well established [6]. On the contrary, there has been limited diffusion of minimally invasive major hepatectomies and it is commonly confined to high volume specialised centres [7]. This is in part due to the more complex anatomical and technical challenges of major hepatic resections, and the inherent limitations of laparoscopic surgery.

Traditional laparoscopic surgery is the most commonly used MIS technique for liver resections whilst there is also an increment in the number of series of robotic liver surgery [8]. Advantages of robotic surgery when compared to traditional laparoscopic surgery are well described and include: a magnified three dimensional (3D) view, tremor filtration and improved dexterity with articulated instruments providing seven degrees of freedom [9]. It also adds some surgeon's specific advantages in terms of ergonomics with the suggested, but not proven, potential reduction of fatigue, increase precision and longer work expectancy. However controversies around robotic surgery remain when compared with laparoscopic surgery. Main limitation was always the higher cost without any evidence suggesting clinical superiority when compared to laparoscopic surgery. There is, in fact to date, lack of agreement whether they should be compared against each other, or directly compared to open surgery. We are of the opinion that both should be grouped as MIS and promoted equally for the benefit of the patient.

In this chapter we describe the key aspects of robotic hepatobiliary surgery, with a focus on technical descriptions, the current evidence base, limitations, and possible future developments.

## 2. Technique

Robotic liver surgery has probably evolved from laparoscopic liver surgery and therefore it is easy to find some similarities. It is however a very different intervention, specially around the economy of movements, and it will vary significantly between centres and surgeons. Local expertise, surgeon's preferences and patient's specific conditions may modify the standard approach but there are some common principles. It is important to mention that currently all reported series have performed this type of intervention with the platform Da Vinci Robot from INTUITIVE® and some of the described technical aspect may apply only to this robotic system. New development of alternative robotic system may bring different technical concepts but the principles will prevail.

### 2.1 Set up and docking

There is significant overlap in the patient positioning, set up and operative technique between laparoscopic and robotic liver resections. This is commonly decided by the operating surgeon and based on his/her preferences. The main difference for a robotic approach is around port placement and the position of the "bed-side"/ assisting surgeon. It is essential to consider instrument clashing when deciding port placement. Alternatives to patient's position include supine (with or without split legs) or left prone position. The latter is the preferred position in some centres to intervene in right posterior segments. Ports position in laparoscopic surgery is more versatile whilst robotic surgery demands wider space between trocars without any port caudal or cephalic to another one (commonly smooth curved line or zig-zag) (**Figures 1–3**).

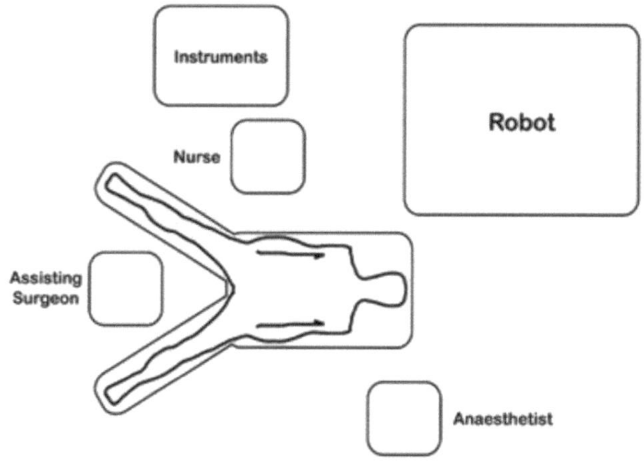


**Figure 1.**
*Patient (supine with split legs in a 15-0 degree reverse Trendelenburg) & assistant (between legs) positioning commonly utilised for major robotic hepatectomy. Subsequent camera and port placement depends on type of resection (**Figures** 2 and 3).*

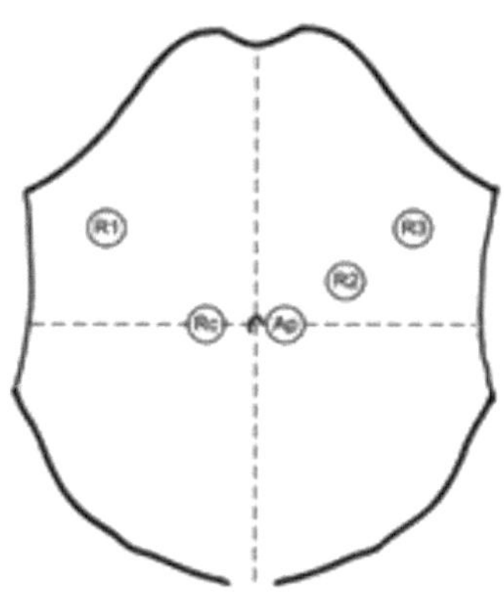


**Figure 2.**
*Port placement for robotic major hepatectomy.*

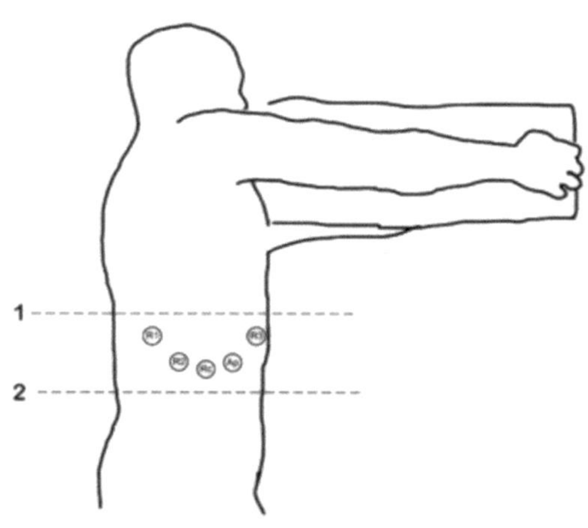


**Figure 3.**
*Patient positioning (left lateral decubitus) & port placement for robotic partial hepatectomy of postero-superior segments. Rc, Robotic Camera Port; Ap, Assistant port (12mm); R1-3, Robotic ports (8-10 mm); 1, transpyloric plane; 2, intertubercular plane.*

Following patient positioning and port insertion, the robotic cart is positioned within the surgical field and the arms docked. Traditional bed-side units are placed cephalic to the surgical field for most hepatobiliary and upper gastro-intestinal procedures. Newer versions allow the cart to be docked sideways to the patient. This adds the benefit of better access to the patient's airway for the anaesthetic team. Irrespective of the system, close collaboration with the anaesthetist is essential at the time of docking.

### 2.2 Liver mobilisation

Following successful docking, the procedural steps are the same as for any hepatic resection and depend on the nature of the required procedure. Liver mobilisation is typically the first step and can be performed utilising a combination of a diathermy or an alternative energy device. For full mobilisation, all liver ligaments (Round/Falciform, Coronary and Triangular) need to be transected. Limited resections however, would not require full mobilisation. Traction and counter traction through lifting of the required liver lobes is provided with the combination of retractors and changes in the patient's position. This requires special attention if the operating table's movement are not linked to the robotic cart. New docking might be required. Lack of tactic feedback can lead to underestimation of the pressure applied to the liver with the consequent capsular tear. Alternatives will include a laparoscopic liver retractor manipulated by the bed side surgeon. Similarly, intraoperative ultrasound can be performed at this point with the close collaboration of the console and bed side surgeons.

### 2.3 Hilar dissection and hepatoduodenal clamping

Robotic surgery can overcome the limitations of laparoscopic surgery during complex hilar dissections, with the combination of 360 degrees angulation, 3D view and scaled movements providing significant advantages to the operator. The exact technicality of hilar dissection will again depend on the surgeon's experience and preferences. Some centres will routinely establish a window in the lesser omentum and pass a sloop or tape to facilitate a Pringle manoeuvre. Similarly to traditional LLS, this can be performed purely intracorporeally or extracorporeally (exteriorization of the clamp/tourniquet via an accessory port). However the high volume specialist centres have suggested this is not routinely required during robotic hepatectomy [10–12].

### 2.4 Parenchymal transection

There are multiple techniques for parenchymal transection and they are widely modified to the personal preferences of the operating surgeon. Kellyclasia technique (clamp-crushing) is held as the current gold standard, although recent advances have focused on the introduction of open and laparoscopic energy devices aimed at reducing blood loss during parenchymal division [13]. This crucial part of the operation is viewed as one of the limiting factors in the diffusion of MIS for the liver across hepatobiliary centres. Whilst robotic surgery improves the suturing capacity and bleeding control in difficult circumstances, the lack of an equivalent robotic energy device may require a hybrid approach with the assisting surgeon performing laparoscopic parenchymal transection at the operating table using an appropriate energy device [14]. Based on this principle, traditional laparoscopic instruments and stapling devices can be used similarly to the traditional laparoscopic approach (i.e. stapling hepatic veins or hilar structures).

### 2.5 Specimen extraction

There is no difference between robotic and laparoscopic surgery at this point, with removal of the specimen via a retrieval bag is achieved following undocking of the robotic arms. Options for specimen extraction include extension of an existing port site or a new incision. There is little evidence comparing all available options but there seems to be a preference towards the Pfannestiel incision [15].

## 3. Current evidence

### 3.1 Major resections

Major hepatectomies (resection of 3 or more contiguous segments) and extended hepatectomies with bile duct resections are complex, challenging procedures. High volume specialist centres have shown a minimally invasive approach to be feasible but the results from the only prospective randomised trial (ORANGE-II plus) are yet to be published [8, 10, 16]. At present, less than 10% of major liver resections are performed laparoscopically, largely due to the challenges posed by the location of the liver, its proximity to major vasculature and the difficulty in appreciating the complex biliary and hepatic vascular anatomy during a laparoscopic procedure [17]. Utilising a robotic approach may negate these disadvantages, with improved views and dexterity facilitating a precise hilar and hepatocaval dissection, advanced suturing and easier biliary-enteric anastomosis.

Specialised centres have published favourable outcomes (**Table 1**) and a limited number of multi centre comparative studies have demonstrated positive results [18–21]. A recent review of outcomes from 584 major robotic liver resections demonstrated acceptable blood loss, operation time, R0 resection rate, length of hospital stay and post op morbidity. When directly compared to laparoscopy, robotic major hepatectomies demonstrated significantly improved rates of post-operative

| Author | Year | Total Cases | Specific procedures | Conversion Rate | Length of stay | Morbidity Rate | Mortality Rate |
|---|---|---|---|---|---|---|---|
| Giulianotti et al. | 2011 | 27 | RH (74%), LH (19%), RTS (7%) | 3.7% | 7 days | 30% | 0% |
| Choi et al. | 2012 | 20 | RH (30%), LH (70%) | 10% | 15 days | 40% | 0% |
| Spampinato et al. | 2014 | 25 | RH (64%), LH (28%), ERH (4%), LLS + SgVI (4%) | 4% | 8 days | 16% | 0% |
| Fruscione et al. | 2019 | 57 | RH (35%), LH (35%), other (30%) | NA – excluded from analysis | 4 days | 28% | 0% |
| Wang et al. | 2019 | 92 | RH (48%), LH (52%) | 1% | 7 days | 13% | 0% |

*RH, right hemi-hepatectomy; LH, left hemi-hepatectomy; RTS, right tri-sectionectomy; ERH, extended right hemi-hepatectomy; LLS, left lateral secitonectomy; SgVII, segment 6. Morbidity rate, includes post op complications from Clavien Dindo grades I-V. Mortality rate, 30 day post-operative mortality.*

**Table 1.**
*Published series focused on outcomes following robotic major hepatectomies in the literature.*

critical care admission, 90 day re-admission rate and a similar length of stay and complication rate [22].

The robotic approach has also been shown to be feasible for simultaneous resection of a colorectal primary malignancy and the associated liver metastasis. Analysis of a small number of major hepatic resection with synchronous colorectal resection, demonstrated robotic resection to have acceptable morbidity and oncological outcomes [23].

The robotic approach has also been considered as an alternative to open surgery for hepatectomies requiring more extended resections and or biliary reconstructions. Outcomes published by 2 specialist centres demonstrated the robotic approach as a safe and feasible alternative to open surgery for hilar cholangiocarcinoma. However whilst technically feasible and safe, the results did not demonstrate equivalence to open surgery. Indeed they reported longer operative times and a higher estimated blood loss relative to open surgery. Furthermore, robotic resection was associated with poorer oncological outcomes with a lower recurrence free survival rate [24, 25].

Given the relative infancy of robotic innovation within the field of minimally invasive surgery, it is perhaps unsurprising that the literature around major robotic liver surgery is somewhat limited. The utility of a laparoscopic approach to major hepatectomy is only presently under investigation and any advantages relative to open surgery remains unestablished. Within this context, it is unclear if open or laparoscopic surgery should be the standard against which robotic surgery is held. At present, level II and III evidence suggests that robotic surgery is safe, feasible, and certainly non inferior to laparoscopic or open surgery. However it remains uncertain if this will translate to clinically significant short and long term outcomes in larger, prospective studies.

### 3.2 Minor resections

Minor hepatic resections, a category encompassing non-anatomical wedge resections, left lateral sectionectomies, segmentectomies and bisegmentectomies, are the most commonly performed minimally invasive hepatic operative interventions in both the laparoscopic and robotic settings [10, 17].

While the evidence discussed above suggests the multitude of technical advantages as well as non-inferiority of the robotic approach to major hepatic resections, it is pertinent to critically examine the role of robotic surgery in minor resections if aiming to confer improved operative outcomes to the greatest number of patients.

In keeping with the increasing trend for parenchymal sparing liver resection, non-anatomical and anatomical wedge resections are the mostly commonly performed robotic liver minor resection [10]. Indeed, a minimal access approach to resect only small amounts of hepatic tissue seems logical considering the morbidity associated with large abdominal incision; a position supported by international consensus in 2008 [26]. Particular difficulties exist, however, when performing laparoscopic in the postero-superior segments of the liver where a combination of the costal margin and rigidity of laparoscopic instruments conspire to make operative access difficult [12].

A number of robotic minor resection cases series from enthusiast centres report broadly equivalent operative times, operative blood loss and post-operative morbidity without significant differences to laparoscopic approaches, although the technical benefit of the robotic endo-articulated wrists were repeatedly emphasised as a partial solution to the difficulties involved with postero-superior segment resections [10, 20, 27, 28]. Furthermore, the use of robotic tremor filtration and gain reduction adjustments were reported to facilitate a greater degree of parenchymal sparing surgery and finer hilar or hepato-caval dissection, technical feats which can be challenging in the laparoscopic setting, potentially reducing requirement for conversion to open [27, 29]. These studies are retrospective, and while some include propensity score matching, prospective randomised controlled trial data is lacking. Results from the Dutch ORANGE-SEGMENTS trial investigating the role of open vs. laparoscopic postero-superior liver segmental resection and results are awaited, but to date no such trials are ongoing in regard to robotic non-anatomical and anatomical wedge resections.

Left lateral sectionectomy consists of the resection of hepatic segments II and III. The minimally invasive approach has become standard of care for this minor resection with comparative ease of access to the left lateral section, a relatively distant relationship to major vasculature and often minimal difficult mobilisation requirement leading this hepatic resection to be considered one of the more straight forward minor hepatectomies [7].

A small number of retrospective studies have aimed to compare the laparoscopic to open approach in left lateral sectionectomy [30–32]. These studies compared a small number of robotic left lateral sectionectomies with retrospective laparoscopic approaches, finding broadly similar results, with no significant differences in operative blood loss, clinical outcomes or operative time, although increased operative costs. A further study, which examined a subgroup of more complex left lateral sectionectomy, with BMI >30, larger tumours or closure operative proximity to major vasculature, reported a significant reduction in operative blood loss, although no significant difference in the overall study group [33]. These results led authors to conclude that the laparoscopic approach to left lateral sectionectomy should remain the standard of care, although it is notable that while gold standard, the only randomised controlled trial comparing laparoscopic vs. open left lateral sectionectomy, ORANGE-II, failed to show a significant difference in outcome when compared the laparoscopic to open approach to left lateral sectionectomy [34]. This result was, in part, due to premature trial cessation due to slow trial recruitment, perhaps reflecting the board uptake of minimal access approach to left lateral sectionectomy. It remains possible that with evidence of clinical non-inferiority of robotics, enthusiastic uptake may further popularise the robotic approach in a similar fashion.

## 4. Oncological outcomes

Given that liver resections are predominantly carried out for malignant pathology, oncological standards such as resection margins, lymph node yields, recurrence and disease free survival are the critical outcomes against which robotic hepatectomy should be evaluated. To that end, we have recently published a review of the literature and found robotic liver surgery to be equivalent with regards to the completeness of the resection margin (96% R0) [35]. Although there are a limited number of studies reporting longer term oncological outcomes such as recurrence and disease free survival, the results so far have been promising.

### 4.1 Hepatocellular carcinoma (HCC)

HCC is the predominant malignancy for which a robotic approach has been utilised, with 40% of the cases published in the literature indicating this as the underlying indication [22]. Three studies have examined the longer term oncological outcomes following robotic hepatectomy in this cohort and found the oncological outcomes to be comparable. Two of these studies compared robotic surgery to open resection and reported a similar 3 year disease free rate at 64% (Lim et al) and

72% (Chen et al). The overall 3 year survival rate was approximately 98% and 93% [36, 37]. The remaining study compared the oncological outcomes between robotic and laparoscopic resections and reported the 5 year disease free and overall survival rate at 42% and 65% respectively [5].

### 4.2 Colorectal liver metastases (CRLM)

Seven studies have examined the oncological outcomes from robotic hepatectomy for colorectal liver metastases. A 100% R0 resection rate was reported by 5 of the 7, whilst the remaining 2 studies reported a rate of 92% and 73.7% [23, 38–43]. A single study evaluated longer term oncological outcomes, and in a propensity matched comparison to laparoscopic resections, reported equivalent 5 year disease free and overall survival rates at 38% and 61% respectively [43]. Matched comparisons of long term oncological outcomes between open and robotic surgery are awaited.

### 4.3 Cholangiocarcinoma (CAA)

Minimally Invasive Surgery utilising a robotic approach should theoretically convey the significant advantages to hilar CCA resections given the necessity of extreme precision and micro-anastomosis formation. However CCA resections form less than 10% of robotic liver surgery in the current literature, likely due to the required tertiary level of surgical expertise and robotic technology [22]. As such, the literature exploring oncolocological outcomes is very limited. The largest case series (48 patients) of patients undergoing robotic resections for Type I, II and III CCA, reported successful lymphadenectomy from stations 7,8,9, 12 and 13 and an R0 resection rate of 72.9% [44]. A single study has reported on longer term outcomes following robotic resections and demonstrated significantly higher rates of recurrence and peritoneal disease when compared to a contemporaneous group of open resections in the same centre [45]. As such whilst technically feasible and safe in expert hands, further studies are required to fully elucidate the oncological equivalence of robotic MIS for CCA.

### 4.4 Gallbladder Cancer

When compared to open radical cholecystectomy, the robotic approach has been shown to result in analogous operative times, blood loss, and length of stay. Specialist centres have also reported equivalent lymph node yields and demonstrated the feasibility of complete robotic lymphadenectomy of stations 8,9 12 and 13 [46–48]. An 100% R0 resection rate has been reported by the only 2 studies that present oncological outcomes [47, 48]. To date, no studies have yet to report on longer term oncological data following robotic radical cholecystectomy.

## 5. Limitations

As with other subspecialties of surgery, while the robotic approach can confer major operative advantages, limitations also exist and it is important to consider these closely, not only for assessment of robotic feasibility, but also in order to adopt adoptions of solutions to such limitations.

The initial purchase of robotic systems poses a major financial outlay to healthcare institutions. With many health systems facing unprecedented pressures, such upfront costs may be difficult to meet. Ongoing maintenance and updates to newer robotic models, as well as requirement for further robotic systems associated with a growing surgical evidence base will add to financial expense.

Such upfront costs may make the financial case for initial investments difficult in a publicly funded health care system such at the UK National Health Service. However, as with all technology, costs of equipment have already been seen to decrease in older models, while newer designs remain at the top of the market. In the same way that laparoscopic stacks and equipment, initially considered a major investment, are now considered as standard in any theatres inventory (albeit with differing quality across healthcare institutions) robotic theatre systems are likely to become common place in the operating theatre complex.

Furthermore, while the earliest days of robotic surgery, saw one company at the forefront of robotic design and technology, maintain a virtual monopoly on the robotic equipment, market competitors have already emerged, a trend which looks set to continue. This is highly likely to bring about a reduction in costs. In this context however, it cannot be assumed that an evidence base for robotic surgery built on one robotic system is necessarily transferable to different systems, and care must be taken when applying this evidence and making financial decisions regarding newer market technology.

In a manner not dissimilar to the initial uptake of laparoscopic minimally invasive surgery in the twentieth century, the uptake of robotic surgery within hepatobiliary surgery has not been as marked as within other surgical specialties. However, this may confer an advantage in financial terms, where robots already purchased and present in theatres based on an early uptake in other specialties can be utilised for education and training in less robotically advanced surgical specialities.

Another disadvantage posed in much of the literature, in both major and minor liver resections is increased operative time, although the clinical maxim "surgical time in measured in inpatient days, not theatre minutes" may be prescient here. Whilst theatre time is a precious financial resource, particularly in an era of unprecedented surgical waiting lists, reduced critical care and overall inpatient stays could confer an overall institutional financial advantage.

Length of surgical theatre time is multifactorial. Technical learning curves of individual surgeons, which have previously shown to be flatter than that of laparoscopic surgery, show operating times inversely proportion to training and experience, as expected with any new skill set [49]. Furthermore, overall operating theatre time not only encompasses the primary surgical procedure, but also robotic system set up, patient positioning, robot docking, and additional tasks performed by the theatre team as a whole. In a similar fashion to the primary surgeon activity discussed above, the increased experience of adequately trained and well drilled theatre team can be expected to significantly reduced theatre times, allowing an increased case load for theatre lists.

While every surgical speciality performs unique technical tasks requiring specific equipment, liver surgery, to perhaps a greater extent than other forms of abdominal surgery, utilise a cornucopia of specific tools not common to other subspecialties. Ultrasonic probes, used for intra operative identification of specific lesion, hepatobiliary specific energy devices and minimally invasive articulated retractors, as well as ultrasonic surgical aspirators, which allow cavitation and aspiration of hepatocytes whilst sparing vascular and biliary structures, are not yet incorporated into standard robotic systems. This technology, however, already exists within the minimal access domain of laparoscopic surgery, so incorporation into robotic systems should not pose an insurmountable barrier.

An often described limitation of MIS is the relative lack of tactile feedback present in open surgery, making dissection of difficult but vital structures significantly more challenging, with potential for catastrophic tissue damage from excessive forces. While much comment was made on this in the advent of laparoscopic surgery, the degree of tactile feedback offered in early robotic surgery systems was even less. Hydraulic haptic feedback systems are, however, already in development with in vivo trials showing significant grip strength reduction more akin to that in open surgery [50, 51].

As with any novel surgical technology, it is necessary to temper adoption of technology with strict clinical governance to maximise patient safety. This includes inclusion of robotics cases in morbidity and mortality discussions, a forum for discussing serious untoward events and near misses, and strategies within scientific literature to avoid publication bias.

Obesity has become an epidemic in many parts of the western world and extremes of BMI offer difficulties in many aspects of surgical practice. While a number of studies in other surgical subspecialties have shown the robotic approach not to offer significantly worsened outcomes in extremes of BMI, hepatobiliary surgery offers specific challenges with non alcoholic fatty liver disease, steatohepatitis and liver cirrhosis associated with morbid obesity [52–54].

A recently published US study examined the effects of BMI, prospectively observing outcomes in patient subgroups of BMIs <25, 25-35 and > 35, found no significant differences found in operative blood loss, operative time of length of stay [55]. With a relatively small number of patients in this study however, more work is required to accurately identify the possible difficulties or benefits posed with hepatic robotic surgery in the obese patient cohort.

Operative training is a vital part of any health service in order to provide future surgeons adequate experience and competence to take on standard as well as challenging cases with a minimal access approach. While early adopters of robotic surgery are often consultant surgeons with strong minimal access laparoscopic practice, for these enthusiasts to become robotic trainers themselves takes time for building of robotic experience. It is therefore expected that robotic training for surgeons in formal training stages will take time to diffuse down, as with the uptake of any new surgical practice. However, flatter learning curves with robotic surgery, with dual operator consoles and built-in simulation trainer modules to robotic surgical systems can offer clinical and non-clinical based training experience. These opportunities will increase with a corresponding increasing prevalence of robotic systems within healthcare institutions.

## 6. Future outlook

While limitations within robotic hepatic surgery exist, the future outlook for incorporation of robotics into liver surgery, with additional integration of other technology offers exciting promise.

Robotics systems, with the primary operator working from a non-sterile station with a visual screen, already offers the opportunity to consult pre-operative imaging for comparison to intra operative findings. Infrared fluorescence technology, incorporated into robotics systems, offers visualisation of vital biliary and vascular structures with near fluorescence of indocyanin green. This poses a major advantage during dissection of the liver hilar structures, where anatomical variation is commonplace and iatrogenic injury can prove catastrophic. With constantly improving imaging and artificial intelligence technology, it is not difficult to imagine intraoperative overlay of imaging to on screen anatomical structures allowing real-time surgical decision making, such as lymph node dissection or surgical resection margins. With the rise of artificial intelligence integrated into robotic systems, it is possible that pre-operative structural recognition of vital hepatobiliary structures or predefined areas within resection margins could be predefined as "no go areas" during operative intervention offering intraoperative artificial intelligence guidance to the operating surgeon. It is perhaps even conceivable that automated robots could perform hepatic resections, with the primary surgeon adopting a supervisory role.

While questions are understandably raised regarding the early stages of surgical training on robotic systems, telecommunications incorporated into robotic systems can arguably vastly improve training in the latter stages. With shared access, real time intra-operative images could be viewed on technology outside of the operating theatres allowing recommendations from experienced colleagues in the event of intraoperative uncertainty. Indeed, it is conceivable the operative control could be managed at work-stations distant to the immediate operating theatre.

Perhaps the most important aspect of the future of robotic surgery, however, will be widespread inclusion into standard surgical practice. If robotic surgery is to exist outside of a few specialist centres, a balance must be struck between using robotics for the most complex technical cases, where a clear evidence base exists within the literature, and the everyday use of the robotic system, allowing not only the operating surgeon but also whole team to become at home managing and trouble-shooting issues that arise with all technology. While major advantages of routine use of robotic technology for, for example, minimally invasive cholecystectomy will be difficult to evidence, adoption of such technology on a day-to-day basis will be essential for surgical training.

## 7. Conclusion

Robotic liver surgery is rapidly evolving. There is growing evidence suggesting this approach to be feasible and safe. This evidence however is limited to highly specialised centres and cannot be consider standard of care. Robotic liver surgery shares the advantages of laparoscopic liver surgery and both should be developed in parallel to promote wider access to minimally invasive surgery for patients undergoing liver resections. Certain limitations remain whilst there is a promising future of innovation and research for robotic liver surgery.

## Author details

Mushfique Alam, Robert Young and Rafael Diaz-Nieto*
Hepatobiliary Surgery Unit, Liverpool University Hospital, Liverpool, United Kingdom

*Address all correspondence to: rafael.diaz-nieto@liverpoolft.nhs.uk

## References


[1] Petrowsky H, Fritsch R, Guckenberger M et al. Modern therapeutic approaches for the treatment of malignant liver tumours. Nature Reviews Gastroenterology & Hepatology. 2020: 17, 755-772

[2] Eskander MF, Bliss LA, Yousafzai OK et al. A nationwide assessment of outcomes after bile duct reconstruction. HPB (Oxford). 2017; 17(9):753-762

[3] Heinrich S & Lang H. Evidence of minimally invasive oncological surgery of the liver. Chirurg (German). 2021; 92(4): 316-325

[4] Xie S-M, Xiong J-J, Liu X-T et al. Laparoscopic versus open liver resection for colorectal liver metastases: A comprehensive systematic review and meta-analysis. Nature Scientific Report. 2017; 7: 1012

[5] Xiangfei M, Yinzhe X, Yingwei P et al. Open versus laparoscopic hepatic resection for hepatocellular carcinoma: a systematic review and meta-analysis. Surg Endosc. 2019; 33(8) 2396-2418

[6] Wakabayashi G, Cherqui D, Geller DA et al. Recommendations for laparoscopic liver resection: A report from the second international consensus conference held in Morioka. Ann Surg 2015; 261: 4

[7] Wang X, Hu M, Zhao Z et al. An improved surgical technique for pure laparoscopic left hemihepatectomy: Ten years experience in a tertiary centre. J Laparoendosc Adv Surg Tech 2016; 26(11): 862-869.

[8] Liu R, Liu Q & Wang Z. Worldwide diffusion of robotic approach in general surgery. Updates in Surgery. 2021; 73:795-797

[9] Roh HF, Nam SH & Kim JM. Robot-assisted laparoscopic surgery versus conventional laparoscopic surgery in randomized controlled trials: A systematic review and meta-analysis. PLoS One 2018; 23:13

[10] Giulianotti PC, Bianco FM, Daskalaki D et al. Robotic liver surgery: technical aspects and review of the literature. HepatoBiliary Surg Nutr 2016;5(4):311-321

[11] Tranchart H, Ceribelli C, Ferretti S, et al. Traditional versus robot-assisted full laparoscopic liver resection: a matched-pair comparative study. World J Surg 2014;38:2904-9. 39.

[12] Casciola L, Patriti A, Ceccarelli G, et al. Robot-assisted parenchymal-sparing liver surgery including lesions located in the posterosuperior segments. Surg Endosc 2011;25:3815-3824.

[13] Pamecha V, Gurusamy KS, Sharma D et al. Techniques for liver parenchymal transection: a meta-analysis of randomised controlled trials. HPB. 2009; 11:275-281

[14] Thakkar R, Kanwar A, Alessandri G et al. Techniques of hepatic transection in robotic surgery – is there still scope for improvement. Advanced Research in Gastroenetrology & Hepatology. 2018; 10(2)

[15] Guilbaud T, Feretti C, Holowko W et al. Laparoscopic Major Hepatectomy: Do not Underestimate the Impact of Specimen Extraction Site. World J Surg. 2020; 44(4): 1223-1230

[16] Masastricht University Medical Centre. The ORANGE II PLUS - Trial: Open Versus Laparoscopic Hemihepatectomy. Found online: The ORANGE II PLUS - Trial: Open Versus Laparoscopic Hemihepatectomy - Full Text View - ClinicalTrials.gov

[17] Nguyen KT, Gamblin TC, Geller DA. World review of laparoscopic liver

resection-2,804 patients. Ann Surg 2009; 250(5): 831-841.

[18] Giulianotti PC, Coratti A, Sbrana F, et al. Robotic liver surgery: results for 70 resections. Surgery 2011;149:29-39

[19] Spampinato MG, Coratti A, Bianco L, et al. Perioperative outcomes of laparoscopic and robot-assisted major hepatectomies: an Italian multi-institutional comparative study. Surg Endosc 2014;28:2973-2979

[20] Tsung A, Geller DA, Sukato DC, et al. Robotic versus laparoscopic hepatectomy: a matched comparison. Ann Surg 2014;259:549-555

[21] Choi GH, Choi SH, Kim SH, et al. Robotic liver resection: technique and results of 30 consecutive procedures. Surg Endosc 2012;26:2247-2258

[22] Ruzzenente A, Alaimo L, Conci S et al. Robotic Liver Surgery: literature review and current evidence. Mini-invasive Surg 2020;4:91

[23] Navarro J, Rho SY, Kang I, Choi GH, Min BS. Robotic simultaneous resection for colorectal liver metastasis: feasibility for all types of liver resection. Langenbecks Arch Surg 2019;404:895-908

[24] Li J, Tan X, Zhang X, et al. Robotic radical surgery for hilar cholangiocarcinoma: a single-centre case series. Int J Med Robot 2020;16:e2076.

[25] Xu Y, Wang H, Ji W, et al. Robotic radical resection for hilar cholangiocarcinoma: perioperative and long-term outcomes of an initial series. Surg Endosc 2016;30:3060-3070

[26] Buell JF, Cherqui D, et al; World Consensus Conference on Laparoscopic Surgery. The international position on laparoscopic liver surgery: The Louisville Statement, 2008. Ann Surg. 2009 Nov;250(5):825-830.

[27] Casciola L, Patriti A, et al. Robot-assisted parenchymal-sparing liver surgery including lesions located in the posterosuperior segments. Surg Endosc. 2011 Dec;25(12):3815-3824.

[28] Giulianotti PC, Coratti A, et al. Robotic liver surgery: results for 70 resections. Surgery. 2011 Jan;149(1):29-39.

[29] Troisi RI, Patriti A, et al.. Robot assistance in liver surgery: a real advantage over a fully laparoscopic approach? Results of a comparative bi-institutional analysis. Int J Med Robot. 2013 Jun;9(2):160-166

[30] Packiam V, Bartlett DL, et al. Minimally invasive liver resection: robotic versus laparoscopic left lateral sectionectomy. J Gastrointest Surg. 2012 Dec;16(12):2233-2238.

[31] Kim JK, Park JS, et al Robotic versus laparoscopic left lateral sectionectomy of liver. Surg Endosc. 2016 Nov;30(11):4756-4764

[32] Lee KF, Cheung YS, et al. Laparoscopic and robotic hepatectomy: experience from a single centre. ANZ J Surg. 2016 Mar;86(3):122-126

[33] Hu M, Liu Y, et al. Robotic versus laparoscopic liver resection in complex cases of left lateral sectionectomy. Int J Surg. 2019 Jul;67:54-60.

[34] E M Wong-Lun-Hing, R M van Dam et al. Randomized clinical trial of open versus laparoscopic left lateral hepatic sectionectomy within an enhanced recovery after surgery programme (ORANGE II study). Br J Surg. 2017 Apr;104(5):525-535.

[35] Diaz-Nieto R, Vyas S, Sharma D et al, Robotic Surgery for Malignant Liver Disease: Systematic Review of Oncological and Surgical Outcomes. Indian Journal of Surgical Oncology. 2019; 11: 565-572

[36] Lim C, Salloum C, Tudisco A, et al. Short- and long-term outcomes after robotic and laparoscopic liver resection for malignancies: a propensity score-matched study. World J Surg 2019;43:1594-1603

[37] Chen PD, Wu CY, Hu RH, et al. Robotic versus open hepatectomy for hepatocellular carcinoma: a matched comparison. Ann Surg Oncol 2017;24:1021-1028

[38] Guerra F, Guadagni S, Pesi B, et al. Outcomes of robotic liver resections for colorectal liver metastases. A multi-institutional analysis of minimally invasive ultrasound-guided robotic surgery. Surg Oncol 2019;28:14-18.

[39] Araujo RLC, Sanctis MA, Barroti LC, Coelho TRV. Robotic approach as a valid strategy to improve the access to posterosuperior hepatic segments-case series and review of literature. J Surg Oncol 2020;121:873-80. 55.

[40] Dwyer RH, Scheidt MJ, Marshall JS, Tsoraides SS. Safety and efficacy of synchronous robotic surgery for colorectal cancer with liver metastases. J Robot Surg 2018;12:603-6. 56

[41] Lin Q, Ye Q, Zhu D, et al. Comparison of minimally invasive and open colorectal resections for patients undergoing simultaneous R0 resection for liver metastases: a propensity score analysis. Int J Colorectal Dis 2015;30:385-395

[42] Guadagni S, Furbetta N, Di Franco G, et al. Robotic-assisted surgery for colorectal liver metastasis: a single-centre experience. J Minim Access Surg 2019;16:160-165

[43] Beard RE, Khan S, Troisi RI, et al. Long-term and oncologic outcomes of robotic versus laparoscopic liver resection for metastatic colorectal cancer: a multicenter, propensity score matching analysis. World J Surg 2020;44:887-895

[44] Li J, Tan X, Zhang X, et al. Robotic radical surgery for hilar cholangiocarcinoma: a single-centre case series. Int J Med Robot 2020;16:e2076

[45] Xu Y, Wang H, Ji W, et al. Robotic radical resection for hilar cholangiocarcinoma: perioperative and long-term outcomes of an initial series. Surg Endosc 2016;30:3060-3070

[46] Shen BY, Zhan Q, Deng XX, et al. Radical resection of gallbladder cancer: could it be robotic? Surg Endosc 2012;26:3245-3250

[47] Byun Y, Choi YJ, Kang JS, et al. Robotic extended cholecystectomy in gallbladder cancer. Surg Endosc 2020;34:3256-3261

[48] Goel M, Khobragade K, Patkar S, Kanetkar A, Kurunkar S. Robotic surgery for gallbladder cancer: operative technique and early outcomes. J Surg Oncol 2019;119:958-963

[49] O'Connor VV, Vuong B, et al. Robotic Minor Hepatectomy Offers a Favorable Learning Curve and May Result in Superior Perioperative Outcomes Compared with Laparoscopic Approach. Am Surg. 2017 Oct 1;83(10):1085-1088

[50] Abiri A, Pensa J, et al. Multi-Modal Haptic Feedback for Grip Force Reduction in Robotic Surgery. Sci Rep. 2019 Mar 21;9(1):5016

[51] Wottawa, Christopher R et al. "Evaluating tactile feedback in robotic surgery for potential clinical application using an animal model." *Surgical endoscopy* vol. 30,8 (2016): 3198-3209

[52] Eddib A, Danakas A, Hughes S, et al. Influence of Morbid Obesity on Surgical Outcomes in Robotic-Assisted

Gynecologic Surgery. J Gynecol Surg. 2014;30(2):81-86

[53] Wee IJY, Kuo LJ, et al. The impact of robotic colorectal surgery in obese patients: a systematic review, meta-analysis, and meta-regression. Surg Endosc. 2019 Nov;33(11):3558-3566.

[54] Wang SE, Daskalaki D, et al. Impact of Obesity on Robot-Assisted Distal Pancreatectomy. J Laparoendosc Adv Surg Tech A. 2016 Jul;26(7):551-556.

[55] Sucandy I, Attili A, et al. The impact of body mass index on perioperative outcomes after robotic liver resection. J Robot Surg. 2020 Feb;14(1):41-46.

Chapter 3

# Robotic-Assisted Minimally Invasive Surgery in Children

*Mario Navarrete-Arellano*


## Abstract

Currently, minimally invasive surgery (MIS) includes conventional laparo-thoracoscopic surgery and robot-assisted surgery (RAS) or robotic surgery. Robotic surgery is performed with robotic devices, for example the Da Vinci system from Intuitive Surgical, which has a miniaturized camera capable of image magnification, a three-dimensional image of the surgical field, and the instruments are articulated with 7 degrees of freedom of movement, and the surgeon operates in a sitting position at a surgical console near the patient. Robotic surgery has gained an enormous surge in use on adults, but it has been slowly accepted for children, although it offers important advantages in complex surgeries. The areas of application of robotic surgery in the pediatric population include urological, general surgery, thoracic, oncological, and otorhinolaryngology, the largest application has been in urological surgery. There is evidence that robotic surgery in children is safe and it is important to offer its benefits. Intraoperative complications are rare, and the frequency of postoperative complications ranges from 0–15%. Recommendations for the implementation of a pediatric robotic surgery program are included. The future will be fascinating with upcoming advancements in robotic surgical systems, the use of artificial intelligence, and digital surgery.


**Keywords:** robot-assisted surgery, minimally invasive surgery, laparoscopy, thoracoscopy, urological, gastrointestinal, hepatobiliary, thoracic, oncological, digital surgery, children

## 1. Introduction

Pediatric robotic surgery offers unique challenges within this rapidly advancing field. There has been a slow rate of uptake within most pediatric surgical centers around the world due to both finance, and difficulties associated with equipment primarily designed for adults. The ergonomics required for the da Vinci® master–slave-type platform currently challenge the small working space in very small children.

Currently, there are three options for surgical treatment for a wide variety of pathologies in the pediatric population, open surgery (traditional) and MIS, which include: conventional laparo-thoracoscopic surgery and RAS.

Minimally invasive techniques are applicable in more than 60% of abdominal and thoracic operations in children, and according to evidence-based data and ethical principles can be used properly [1].



IntechOpen

In 1994, the first robotic system used in the urological practice known as AESOP was introduced. Later, the evolution of these devices would bring the Zeus system and finally the Da Vinci system while continuously increasing their precision and effectiveness [2].

Since these initial reports, robotic surgery has seen widespread application within the adult population, especially in urologic and gynecologic procedures. As is often the case for new devices, technology, and therapeutic options in surgery, the application of robotic surgery for children has occurred more slowly than in adults. This caution is due in part to technical limitations with developing appropriately sized instruments for the pediatric patient; however, in recent years broader implementation has been seen [3–6].

In April 2001, Meininger et al. [7] published the first cases of RAS in children. The first of these two Nissen fundoplication procedures was reported as occurring in July 2000 [7–10]. Shortly afterward, the first robotic urological procedure in a child was undertaken in March 2002 by Peters et al. (personal communication, July 2002) who performed a pyeloplasty using the da Vinci® [11, 12]. Since then to date, more than 70 different surgical techniques have been published [13, 14].

Currently, the only robotic system that is approved for pediatric use is the da Vinci Surgical System (Intuitive Surgical, Sunnyvale, CA) [7]. The da Vinci robot is well suited for children of all ages, including infants and newborns, using careful preoperative planning, this allows the da Vinci to be used for numerous procedures in small children [14, 15].

The evolution of conventional laparoscopic surgery highlights the transitory stages that follow adoption and diffusion of surgical innovation [16–18]. RAS was introduced to the specialty of pediatric surgery following initial case reports in the early 21st century. Subsequently, this promising surgical technology has undergone a formative 10-year period of introduction, development, early dispersion, exploration and preliminary assessment [13].

Cundy et al. [13], performed a 2013 systematic literature search for all reported cases of RAS in children during an 11-year period. During this time, 2,393 procedures in 1,840 patients were reported and the most prevalent gastrointestinal, genitourinary, and thoracic procedures were fundoplication, pyeloplasty, and lobectomy, respectively.

Due to the limitations of conventional laparoscopic surgery in pediatric patients, expert pediatric surgeons should only perform the more complex or reconstructive laparoscopic techniques [19].

There have been few reports that have been published about robotic general pediatric surgery [20–29]. Thus, far, the largest number of procedures and publications have been produced about robotic urological pediatric surgery [11–13, 30–45]. Trends in the literature indicate that pediatric RAS is continuing to be globally utilized [11, 13, 30–35, 43–46].

The safety of RAS in children is reported to be similar to open procedures, and the outcomes are at least equivalent to conventional laparoscopy [47]. Robotic surgery on smaller children and infants require special considerations when discussing robotic surgery [48].

Numerous case reports, case series, and comparative studies have unequivocally demonstrated that robotic surgery in children is safe [13].

In systematic investigations of databases of pediatric RAS, the global surgical conversion rate was 4.7% [22], and a net overall surgical conversion rate of 2.5% was reported [13]. In published studies of pediatric RAS, transoperative complications are infrequent, and in the postoperative period, the frequency varies from 0 to 15% [22, 49–51].

## 2. Characteristics, advantages, benefits, limitations and applications of robotic surgery

### 2.1 Characteristics

In RAS robotic devices are used, such as the Da Vinci system from Intuitive Surgical, which has a miniaturized camera and the surgeon operates seated at a console close to the patient (telesurgery), with three-dimensional and magnified images of the operative field, and manipulates articulated instruments controlled by their hands and feet; It is supported by a second surgeon positioned next to the patient at the exposure of the operative field, with retraction, suction and exchange of instruments in the arms of the robot. There is greater precision than in open surgery and conventional laparo-thoracoscopic surgery [52].

### 2.2 Advantages

RAS enables more refined hand-eye coordination, superior suturing skills, better dexterity, and precise dissection. It is achieved by the characteristics of robotic surgical platforms that include motion scaling, greater optical magnification, 3D, and stereoscopic vision, increased articulated instrument tip dexterity, tremor filtration, operator-controlled camera movement, and elimination of the fulcrum effect [13], all of this translates into greater safety for patients and advantages for the surgeon.

Robotic instruments were specifically designed to mimic human wrist movements, allow 7 degrees of freedom of movement, and can be particularly advantageous for newborns, infants, and young children, as well as, certain hard-to-reach anatomical areas [29, 46]. By operating seated at the console, surgical fatigue and tremors are reduced [53].

### 2.3 Benefits

Robotic enhancements offer improvements in the technical capacity of human performance for surgery within spatially restricted workspaces in children [13]. Less time is required to acquire the right skills and confidence with RAS, "The learning curve is shorter" [46, 54–56]. Robotic assistance will allow more pediatric surgeons to perform a greater volume of minimally invasive procedures [57].

It also has a real benefit for the pediatric patient in terms of: minimizing operative trauma, minimal scarring, less postoperative pain, less need for opioids, less bleeding and transfusions, fewer complications, less risk of infection, shorter hospitalization, and quick return to daily activities, this also benefits parents [46, 47, 58].

### 2.4 Limitations

There are limitations in RAS, this includes, access to the patient by the anesthesiologist is limited after the robot is docked, changes to patient position or access to the patient requires detachment of the robot, and patients must remain entirely paralyzed when the robot is docked [59].

In addition, RAS frequently requires Trendelenburg or reverse Trendelenburg steeper positioning, which has hemodynamic consequences. This situation can typically be mitigated by adequate volume expansion [60].

Infants are typically more susceptible to the respiratory effects of pneumoperitoneum than older children or adults, abdominal insufflation decreases respiratory compliance and increases airway pressures, and the instilled $CO_2$ can cause hypercapnia and acidosis [61].

The primary disadvantage of robotic surgical technology in pediatric surgery is related to the size of the surgical robot and its associated instruments [4, 5, 46], the robotic instruments are only available in 2 sizes, 8 mm and 5 mm. Similarly, robotic endoscopes (lens) are currently only available as 12.0 mm and 8.5 mm.

The cost analysis for the use of the robot is not strictly measured by numerical cost in dollars, but should be considered as value equating to quality (as defined by positive outcomes/cost). Naturally, there is the initial cost of purchasing and maintaining the robot itself, as well as the increased costs from the disposable robotic equipment and the longer operative times [4]. It should be noted other factors associated with the robotic portion of a procedure, such as increased operating room or anesthesia time, staff training, and cost of marketing campaigns [62].

In contrast, patient and parent satisfaction, as well as emotional and professional benefits, should also be considered when evaluating cost/satisfaction of this type of investment [63]. One study found that it takes at least 3 to 5 cases per week in a program to demonstrate a net gain from robotic surgery [64].

Other cost analyses suggest that robotic surgeries are more expensive than those associated with laparoscopic or open surgery [65, 66]. However, RAS is associated with a 2% decrease in anastomotic leaks [67, 68]. This reduces hospitalization and costs of managing the resulting surgical morbidity, and benefits the earlier return of the patient to the workforce [66]. In addition, by preferably performing difficult and complex cases in which robotic surgery adds value to patient care; it should be a solution with the best profitability in hospitals that have a robotic system. In some countries such as in Latin America, costs represent a great inconvenience for the advancement of robotic surgery in children, especially in private hospitals.

A short hospital stay, prudent use of instruments, reduced operating room times, and competent robotic equipment reduce costs [69]. Therefore, future comparative analyses of outcomes in children should include financial factors such as loss of human capital, parents [70].

### 2.5 Applications

Robotic surgery has been used in almost all pediatric surgical subspecialties, including urology, general surgery (gastrointestinal-hepatopancreatobiliary), thoracic, oncology, and otorhinolaryngology. Among pediatric disciplines, robotic surgery is used most frequently in urology.

The best indications for robotic surgery are procedures that require a small surgical field, fine and precise dissection, and secure intracorporeal sutures [71]. The RAS have special application in complex and reconstructive surgery, for these procedures, from the open technique; surgeons often jump to RAS [14]. RAS in otorhinolaryngology with the application of the transoral approach is particularly useful in masses of the tongue base [72]. Furthermore, RAS has performed a wide spectrum of surgical procedures in children [13].

## 3. Urologic robotic surgery

To date, the application of MIS in pediatric urology has evolved over more than 30 years [73]. Urology has the highest acceptance of robotic surgery within pediatrics. The first use of robotics in children was a pyeloplasty for ureteropelvic junction (UPJ) obstruction, because the ureteropelvic anastomosis was a technical challenge using conventional laparoscopic surgery [11, 12].

In a systematic bibliographic search that was carried out of all the published cases of pediatric robot-assisted urological surgery between 2003 and 2016. A total of 151 publications that reported 3688 procedures in 3372 patients were identified. The most reported procedures were pyeloplasty (1923), ureteral reimplantation (1120), heminephrectomy (136), and nephrectomy or nephroureterectomy (117). There were 16 countries and 48 institutions represented in this literature [6].

We will approach the surgical urological pathology of the child based on the anatomy of the urinary tract as follows, i. Upper urinary tract, ii. Lower urinary tract and iii. Miscellaneous procedures.

### 3.1 RAS on the upper urinary tract

#### *3.1.1 Nephrectomy*

In pediatric patients, complete or partial nephrectomies are indicated more frequently for benign diseases and less frequently for malignant diseases. Indications for RAS nephrectomy for benign diseases are multicystic dysplastic kidney disease, kidney exclusion due to various pathologies, such as UPJ obstruction, reflux nephropathy, among others, indications of malignant tumors, particularly Wilms tumor are increasing legitimizing itself through corresponding treatment protocols, and surgery performed while adhering strictly to oncological surgical rules [74].

In nephrectomy, the initial step is the dissection and exposure of the renal pedicle, its ligation and cutting. The next step, the kidney is completely freed from its surrounding tissue. Subsequently, the dissection of the ureter is performed, in the case of radical nephroureterectomy it should be performed up to the bladder. The kidney is extracted through the umbilical access, in case of nephrectomy due to tumor, the use of a collection bag is mandatory, and it is removed through a Pfannenstiel incision, and finally lymph node sampling is crucial for surgical staging and guiding subsequent treatment.

#### *3.1.2 Partial nephrectomy*

Ureteral duplication is the most common congenital abnormality of the urinary tract. Partial nephrectomy for benign indication is performed for the resection of a deficient or non-functional fraction of a duplex system and can cause or be associated with obstruction and hydronephrosis, dysplasia, megaureter, ureterocele, and vesicoureteral reflux. Heminephroureterectomy is performed in cases with a reflux system [73]. It is recommended before surgery, to place a stent in the ureter to be preserved (for easy identification during dissection). If the ureter of the remaining fraction is to be reimplanted or if an ectopic ureter is to be followed in the deep pelvis, the robot is repositioned between the patient's legs and redocked [75].

#### *3.1.3 Pyeloplasty*

Robot-assisted pyeloplasty is the most common procedure performed robotically in pediatric patients, both within urology and overall [76]. The excellent experience with robot-assisted pyeloplasty has challenged other approaches as a new standard for the treatment of UPJ obstruction.

Dismembered pyeloplasty (Anderson-Hynes) includes resection of the UPJ and reduction of the renal pelvis. In the technique, the ureter is incised and spatulated laterally to provide sufficient ureteral wall length to achieve a wide side-to-side anastomosis. Once the anterior layer of the pelvic-ureteral anastomosis has been sutured, an antegrade transanastomotic double-J stent is passed. J-Vac transabdominal drainage was used in the surgical bed.

Patients undergoing robotic pyeloplasty have a shorter hospital stay, and less need for analgesics; however, there is no difference in the success rate of robotic pyeloplasty in comparison to the other two approaches [77–79].

In robotic pyeloplasty the learning curve is much shorter. This allows some surgeons to transition from the open pyeloplasty to the robotic approach without any prior laparoscopic experience with this technique [80].

Pyeloplasty in infants less than 10 kg has been performed successfully. A multi-institutional study of 60 infants less than 12 months old with a 91% success rate and an 11% complication rate, which is similar to other studies on larger children and adults [81]. The foregoing supports the personal experience of the author.

Also, the retroperitoneal robotic approach is indicated mainly for patients with previous abdominal surgery, when adhesion syndrome is suspected, and it has been validated for pyeloplasty and other techniques in this anatomical area [82].

#### *3.1.4 Ureteroureterostomy*

The procedures performed included pyeloureterostomy for incomplete duplication and lower pole UPJ obstruction and ipsilateral ureteroureterostomy along with distal ureterectomy for obstruction in a dysplastic upper pole with ureteral, ectopia, for the treatment of duplex anomalies and reconstruction of obstructed dilated ureteral segments [83]. This can also be applied to the lower ureter in duplex systems where it helps to avoid reimplantation of disparate ureters in the same tunnel. Also, transperitoneal robotic ureteroureterostomies have been reported for mid ureteric strictures and also for the correction of retrocaval ureters [84, 85]. Also with robotic assistance, the removal of a large ureteric stone at any level with the placement and closure of a stent is a relatively simple affair, using the Mikulicz procedure to close the ureterotomy or a spatulate anastomosis.

#### *3.1.5 Ureterocalicostomy*

Ureterocalicostomy is a potential, and technically feasible option in patients with UPJ obstruction and significant lower pole caliectasis which is often reserved for patients with a failed pyeloplasty and a minimal pelvis, or patients with an exaggerated intrarenal pelvis [86]. An ureterocalicostomy is a procedure in which the ureter is sutured to the lowermost calyx of the kidney. It is a salvage operation, which should be in the arsenal of every surgeon operating the UPJ [87]. The robotic approach is a good option.

### 3.2 RAS on the lower urinary tract

#### *3.2.1 Extravesical ureteral reimplantation*

The most performed procedure in the lower urinary tract in children is the antireflux ureteral reimplantation [13]. Indications for the surgical treatment of pediatric vesicoureteral reflux include severe urinary tract infections while taking continuous antibiotics prophylaxis, renal scarring, and worsening or non-resolution vesicoureteral reflux. Robotic ureteral reimplantation can be done by an extravesical or intravesical approach and, of these approaches, the extravesical is much more widely reported [88, 89]. The extravesical procedure is a ureteral reimplantation according to the well-established technique of Lich-Gregoir, for achieving an antireflux mechanism. This technique is an accepted alternative to endoscopic treatment and open reimplantation techniques in pediatric patients [73]. However, open surgery remains the gold standard for ureteral reimplantation [90].

The long-term results of the antireflux procedure are evaluated in terms of preservation of differential renal function, absence of urinary tract infections, and adequate urinary drainage, with a follow-up of more than one year [91]. In a prospective study of children undergoing robot extravesical ureteral reimplantation at eight academic centers from 2015 to 2017, 143 patients (199 ureters). The majority of ureters (73.4%) had grade III or higher vesicoureteral reflux preoperatively. Radiographic resolution was present in 93.8% of ureters. Robotic ureteral reimplantation should be considered as one of several viable options for management of vesicoureteral reflux in children [92].

#### *3.2.2 Appendico-vesicostomy and continent catheterizable channels*

##### *3.2.2.1 Appendicovesicostomy (Mitrofanoff)*

Complete bladder emptying in children with bladder emptying dysfunction (neuropathic bladder) is achieved with clean intermittent catheterization (CIC). In 1980, Mitrofanoff described his technique of a continent appendicovesicostomy for patients when transurethral CIC cannot be carried out for any reason. When medical therapy fails in the neuropathic bladder, the surgery aims to preserve upper tract function and social continence. A cystostomy with a continent opening easy to catheterize and associated with a closure of the vesical neck, was the objective. The tip of the appendix opened into the bladder at the end of an antireflux submucosal tunnel and the other end hemmed to the skin. The bladder neck is usually closed in the same operation. The continence of the vesicostomy is total and the comfort obtained is excellent [93].

The surgical technique is analogous to the Lich-Gregoir technique, to create an antireflux mechanism. The appendicocutaneostomy can be placed in the umbilicus or in the right lower abdominal quadrant [73]. Robotic continence procedures have been shown to be a safe and effective alternative [94]. An important point is to assess whether a simultaneous bladder augmentation is performed [95].

In patients with neurogenic bowel and bladder secondary to spinal dysraphism who tend to have multiple limb spasms and spinal scoliosis, RAS is a good option [96]. Complex lower urinary tract reconstruction defined as reconstruction of the bladder neck or catheterizable continent ducts, or both, as well as the creation of an antegrade Malone continence enema, for better management of constipation [97].

#### *3.2.3 Augmentation cystoplasty*

Augmentation cystoplasty often performed in the context of other reconstructive procedures such as appendicovesicostomy or bladder neck reconstruction. The procedure of bladder augmentation can be performed using a mega-ureter when nephrectomy is anticipated. At present day, the ileocystoplasty represents the currently accepted standard of care [73]. In robotic technique, a 20 cm segment of ileum is selected and isolated. Intestinal continuity is restored, and in the postoperative, the bladder is drained with a suprapubic tube, a urethral catheter and another catheter through the Mitrofanoff channel [98]. Another tissue option for bladder augmentation is the sigmoid colon, this technique significantly improved urodynamic parameters, such as bladder accommodation and filling pressure in children with myelomeningocele-associated neurogenic bladder [99].

### 3.3 Pediatric urology miscellaneous procedures

The miscellaneous pediatric urology procedures are some surgeries in the pelvic area, a narrow field that is ideal for the robotic approach. There are reports from

RAS of; symptomatic bladder diverticulum excision [36], symptomatic or malignant urachal cyst excision [100], posterior urethral diverticula excision, mainly after surgical reconstruction of imperforate anus [101], prostatic utricle removal, is a malformation due to incomplete regression of Müllerian ducts [102], and varicocele cure, a condition that has a significant association with infertility [103].

## 4. General surgery (gastrointestinal and hepatopancreatobiliary)

RAS in general surgery, and thoracic surgery have not yet reached the magnitude that it has in pediatric urology. Robotic procedures that have been reported include, fundoplication, cholecystectomy, choledochal cysts resection, hepatectomy, colectomies, proctectomy with ileal pouch-anorectal anastomosis [104]. Other techniques are, Thal fundoplication and salpingo-oophorectomy [8], Soave pull-through procedure for Hirschsprung's disease [105]. Others that are less common, RAS for the treatment of duodenal obstruction, such as the Ladd cure in intestinal malrotation, the duodenojejunostomy for superior mesenteric artery syndrome [106], the repair of congenital duodenal atresia [107], and gastroduodenal obstruction due to trichobezoar [14].

Hepatopancreatobiliary RAS in children inevitably involves high complexity, such as Kasai portoenterostomies and choledochal cyst resection [108–109]. Furthermore, liver resection, robot-assisted generally indicated for treatment of tumors [110].

### 4.1 Fundoplication

Fundoplication is the most widely performed and reported robotic-assisted surgery in pediatric general and thoracic surgery [3].

When comparing conventional laparoscopic primary fundoplication and RAS in children, there were no differences between the two groups in terms of operative time, length of hospital stay, conversions, and complications. The conclusion is that RAS is a safe alternative to conventional laparoscopic surgery [111]. Regarding the advantages of RAS, a systematic review of primary fundoplication showed that postoperative complications are reduced in the robotic group. Because in the RAS there is greater dexterity and precision in the subphrenic space, than with laparoscopy [112]. In addition, RAS plays an important role in difficult cases, such as obese patients, large hiatal hernias, and redo fundoplication [113, 114]. On the other hand, with conventional laparoscopy, only skilled pediatric surgeons resolve difficult cases [114].

### 4.2 Choledochal cyst resection

Choledochal cyst resection and reconstructive Roux-en-Y hepaticojejunostomy are technically complex and, only in Southeast Asian centers there is extensive experience in the laparoscopic technique. In the rest of the pediatric centers of the world, most of this surgeries are performed with the open technique [115].

In 2006, the first pediatric RAS choledochal cyst resection was reported [116]. Since that time and up to 2019, several authors have reported cohorts of 1 to 39 pediatric patients undergoing RAS choledochal cyst resection [109]. A recent publication informed 70 cases with RAS and 70 cases by conventional laparoscopy, and concluded that RAS choledochal cyst excision and hepaticojejunostomy were associated with better short-term intraoperative and postoperative outcomes, and proved the safety and feasibility of RAS in children with choledochal cysts [117].

The ideal treatment for children with choledochal cyst, nowadays, is MIS, laparoscopic, through expert pediatric surgeons or RAS, in institutions where technology is available. But, if one or another situation is not present, the author recommends continuing with the open approach to offer children the greatest safety and effectiveness [109].

### 4.3 Kasai procedure

The Kasai procedure can be ideal for RAS because it is a complex technique, it has an ideal instrumentation to dissect the hepatic portal and find the portal plate [118]. To date, there are very few reported cases of Kasai operation for RAS for biliary atresia. The experience is larger with conventional laparoscopy, especially in Southeast Asian countries, where the pathology is more frequent than in other latitudes of the world [115].

### 4.4 Pancreatic pathology

There are very few publications of pancreatic pathology in children treated with RAS, we find only case reports about: tumor enucleation, distal pancreatectomy, subtotal pancreatectomy, and pancreaticoduodenectomy. The traditional open surgeries have been largely replaced by MIS, including laparoscopic surgery and RAS.

RAS distal spleen-sparing pancreatectomy is safe and feasible in pediatric patients with insulinoma [119]. Also, robotic enucleation is indicated in small neuroendocrine tumors of the pancreas. This technique provides the dual benefits of minimal invasiveness and good preservation of the pancreatic parenchyma. The experience has demonstrated the feasibility and safety of the RAS enucleation, with an excellent curative effect for pediatric insulinoma [120, 121].

### 4.5 Soave pull-through

Hirschsprung's disease (HSCR) has also been shown to benefit from robotic surgery, the outcome of totally robotic soave pull-through for HSCR is promising. This technique is particularly suitable for older HSCR patients, even those requiring a redo surgery, and represents a valid alternative for HSCR patients. In cases of total colonic aganglionosis, for the hepatic angle or only recto sigmoid, RAS has been used and its versatility has been confirmed. The published results are promising, continence scored from excellent to good in all patients who could be evaluated in this regard [105]. In the first series of infants less than 6 kg who underwent the Swenson RAS, morbidity did not increase [122].

### 4.6 Treatment of duodenal obstruction

Superior mesenteric artery syndrome is a rare condition that results from intermittent functional obstruction of the third part of the duodenum. The diagnostic criteria are clinical, radiological and endoscopic. The classic approach has been open surgery [123]. There are case reports of robotic Roux-en-Y duodenojejunostomy as a surgical option for the treatment of this condition [106, 124].

Robotic repair of congenital duodenal atresia may help overcome the obstacles presented by the use of traditional rigid laparoscopic instruments, due to the difficulty in constructing a precise duodenal anastomosis, with robotic surgery the procedure is relatively straightforward [107]. About gastroduodenal obstruction due to trichobezoar in children and laparoscopy, we found several reports. We operated with RAS on a 12-year-old girl weighing 23 kg with pica and psychological disorder, with success and without postoperative morbidity [14].

## 4.7 Various procedures in general surgery

### *4.7.1 Cholecystectomy*

Elective robot-assisted cholecystectomy *is* relatively prevalent in the literature [13]. Multiport robotic cholecystectomy and single-site robotic cholecystectomy are the approach options. Robotic cholecystectomy is safe and effective and serves as an excellent introductory procedure for pediatric surgeons considering the development of a pediatric robotic surgery program, useful for training [125].

### *4.7.2 Splenectomy*

Splenectomy remains the mainstay of treatment for the sequelae of pediatric hereditary hematologic disorders. These conditions can lead to splenomegaly, medically refractory cytopenias, and dependence on transfusions. Laparoscopic splenectomy is the standard of surgical care. Robot-assisted splenectomy is an option and is associated with a shorter length of hospital stay compared to laparoscopic splenectomy [126].

### *4.7.3 Gynecological surgery*

There are case reports and series documenting a variety of robotic gynecological surgeries in children with favorable results. Procedures consisted of ovarian cystectomies, oophorectomies for ovarian masses, and salpingo-oophorectomy for gonadal dysgenesis [127]. In addition, robotic resection of mature cystic teratoma and mucinous ovarian tumor. It is an easy and safe technique in selected patients and also for the treatment of complex gynecological diseases [128]. Surgeries in the pelvis have a reduced field of work and are ideal for the robotic approach.

### *4.7.4 Heller's cardiomyotomy for achalasia*

Achalasia is rare in children. Surgical options include open, laparoscopic, and robotic approaches, and Heller's myotomy remains the treatment of choice. Concomitant partial posterior fundoplication is suggested for all patients. Heller's robotic myotomy for esophageal achalasia in children has been shown to be safe and effective. Both laparoscopic and robotic esophageal myotomy are comparable in their results. However, robotic surgery is superior in terms of avoiding mucosal perforation, this complication occurred in 16% of patients in the laparoscopic group [129–131].

### *4.7.5 Management for anorectal malformations*

Anorectal pull-through for anorectal malformations, with the robotic technology assists the pediatric surgeon by increasing dexterity and precision of movement. This is important in anorectal malformations surgery, where the dissection of the fistula and the pull-through of the rectum into the muscular complex are crucial to achieve continence in future. RAS permits easier closure of the fistula, improves reconstruction technique, and minimizes trauma to important surrounding structures, providing better visualization of the muscular complex. Robotic anorectal pull-through makes use of fundamental concepts learned from decades of high-anorectal malformation open repair, and combines them with modern advances in surgical instrumentation and techniques [132].

## 5. Thoracic robotic surgery

The global experience in thoracoscopic surgery in children is more than 30 years compared to robot-assisted thoracic surgery (RATS). The learning curve of thoracoscopy is longer compared to RAS. Thoracic MIS reduces the risk of thoracic and spinal deformities after lung resection in children. Lobectomy is one of the robotic techniques most frequently performed in children [133].

Early publications on RATS in children reported having performed cardiovascular techniques such as patent ductus arteriosus (PDA) closure and vascular ring section [134, 135]. Le Bret, et al. [134] in 2000, 56 children operated on for PDA surgical closure, 28 cases with thoracoscopy and 28 cases with robotic approach. They used the ZEUS robotic surgical system (Computer Motion, Inc., Goleta, CA. USA). Their results were comparable in both approaches.

Cundy et al. [13], in a systematic search in the literature of reported cases of robotic surgery in children of 2393 procedures, thoracic procedures accounted for 3.2% (77 surgeries and 12 different techniques), and the conversion rate was 10% in thoracic procedures. In this report, the five most frequent RATS procedures are: lobectomy (18), thymectomy (14), benign mass excision (9), diaphragmatic plasty (8), and malignant tumor resection (5).

There are three series reported with a greater number of cases, each with 11 RATS in children (total 33), in order of frequency the procedures include: tumor masses resection (8), lobectomy (7), diaphragmatic plication (4), diaphragmatic plasty (3), esophageal atresia correction (3), bronchogenic cysts resection (3) and unique procedures of segmentectomy, esophageal duplication resection, pleural and lung biopsies, gastric tube/esophagoplasty and Heller myotomy. Overall, there were 6 (18%) conversions to open surgery in neonatal patients and (3) 9% postoperative complications. The neonatal thorax represents the greatest obstacle in the adaptation of the 5 or 8 mm robotic platform instruments [20, 133, 136]. In RATS, children weighing more than 4 kg are more easily treated [15].

### 5.1 Pulmonary lobectomy

The most common RATS in children is lobectomy. The first publication on robotic lobectomy, including pediatric cases, was by Park et al. [137], in 2006. Series with few cases of segmental lung resections and lobectomies have been published with excellent results with conversions mainly on the first attempt [14, 15, 133, 136]. Addressing the disadvantages of RATS lobectomy, a prolonged total operative time was reported, but without having a negative effect, since it did not increase the postoperative morbidity and mortality of patients [138].

### 5.2 Congenital diaphragmatic hernia repair

Congenital diaphragm abnormalities, including eventration and Morgagni and Bochdalek diaphragmatic hernias, have been successfully repaired through the use of conventional MIS. However, some reports have shown a high recurrence rate for some defects. Robotic surgery is the alternative to close diaphragmatic hernias more efficiently [139].

Some authors prefer the thoracic approach to repair Bochdalek's diaphragmatic hernia, but infants weighing less than 2.5 kg are better treated with the abdominal approach. The author performed one case of Morgagni's diaphragmatic hernia and another case of Bochdalek's diaphragmatic hernia via the abdominal route. Robotic assistance allows the surgeon to more easily reach this area to suture diaphragmatic defects [139].

Acquired anomalies, such as diaphragmatic paralysis, can also be resolved with RATS [14, 139].

### 5.3 Thymectomy

Radical thymectomy is the comprehensive treatment of myasthenia gravis. The feasibility and effectiveness of robotic thymectomy is evident in this cohort study [140]. In addition, performing the "early thymectomy" (performed within a year of diagnosis) resulted in higher remission rates compared to "late thymectomy" [141], including minimizing the adverse effects of immunosuppression in pediatric patients [142].

In recent studies including 49 children, thoracoscopic thymectomy was also safe for children with juvenile myasthenia gravis (JMG) [143, 144]. Two other studies with 9 and 18 children, reported the same results [145, 146]. Robotic thymectomy is a safe procedure, complications were low, and without mortality. Thymectomy should be offered as a part of multimodal therapy for treating children and adolescents with acetylcholine receptor antibody-Positive JMG [146].

### 5.4 Other robotic thoracic procedures

There are RATS publications of other specific procedures, such as tracheopexy for the treatment of severe tracheomalacia [147], and reports of pediatric cases of resection of a bronchogenic cyst [148, 149].

## 6. Oncologic robotic surgery

Presently, the use of MIS in patients with cancer is progressing. However, the role of MIS in children with solid neoplasms is less clear than it is in adults. Although the use of diagnostic MIS to obtain biopsy specimens for pathology is accepted in pediatric surgical oncology, there is limited evidence to support the use of MIS for the resection of malignancies (solid tumors) in the thorax and abdomen in children [150].

Open surgery remains the main technique for the resection of solid tumors in children. RAS offers technical and ergonomic advantages that can make MIS more achievable in this environment, allowing benefits for both the patient and the surgeon. Reduced postoperative recovery time and faster initiation of adjuvant therapy are the most important benefits for the patient [104].

A systematic search of multiple electronic databases, of 23 publications, reported 40 cancer cases in total. The indications for surgery were more than 20 different pathologies. One third of the tumors were malignant. Most of the procedures involved abdominal or retroperitoneal tumors in adolescent patients. Oncological adverse events were two isolated events, one tumor spillage and one residual disease. The evidence is limited to case reports and small case series only. Pediatric cancer surgery is an area of opportunity for robotic surgery. Its technical challenges create the opportunity to develop robotic approaches that meet the challenges of complex cancer procedures [151].

### 6.1 Thoracic tumors

As an anecdote, the robot appears to be well adapted to complex mediastinal dissection and has been used in excision of left ventricular myxoma [152], and in excision of complex massive leiomyoma of the esophagus [153]. The robot offered excellent visualization and ease of resection. The other case of complex massive retrocardiac esophageal leiomyoma was successfully removed using RAS. In the latter case, intraoperative esophagoscopy and transillumination were useful adjuncts to identify the esophagus and develop a safe extramucosal dissection plane.

There is a publication with five pediatric patients with a mean age of 9.8 years and weight of 41.5 kg, who underwent robotic resection of a mediastinal thoracic mass, including a ganglioneuroma, ganglioneuroblastoma, teratoma, germ cell tumor, and a large inflammatory mass of unclear etiology. The application of RATS in malignant solid tumors in children in selected cases is an option, but oncological surgical principles should be applied [154].

### 6.2 Abdominal tumors

There are mostly individual case reports for robot-assisted abdominal oncological surgery in children.

Neuroblastoma is the most common extracranial solid tumor in children and the most common malignancy in infants. Complete resection is curative in low-stage disease. Robotic surgery can skeletonize abdominal blood vessels in the tumor and cut the tumor into pieces, including stage IV retroperitoneal neuroblastoma [155, 156].

Juvenile cystic adenomyoma is the focal presence of ectopic endometrial glands and stroma within the uterine myometrium. Another case, a 15-year-old adolescent girl underwent RAS of a 4 cm cyst, and the uterus was closed in four layers, the postoperative period was uneventful [157].

Management of rhabdomyosarcoma. A 22-month-old, 8-kg boy with an embryo-rhabdomyosarcoma in the urinary bladder and prostate, the treatment was a robot-assisted radical cystoprostatectomy, and the postoperative course was uneventful [158]. Another application of RAS is in the dissection of retroperitoneal lymph nodes in selected pediatric and adolescent patients with paratesticular rhabdomyosarcoma or germ cell tumor of the testicle, a report of a case of each of these conditions, they were treated with good results. The robotic approach to extended lymph node dissection is suitable [159].

Robotic partial nephrectomy has been reported in appropriately selected children with renal cell carcinoma. However, there are limited reports of laparoscopic or robotic partial nephrectomy for cancer surgery in children. RAS allows for an oncologically sound resection of partial nephrectomy, as well as extended lymph node dissection [160].

Robotic adrenalectomy is an increasingly used procedure in patients with a variety of surgical adrenal lesions, including adenomas, aldosteronomas, pheochromocytomas, and adrenal gland metastases. Emerging literature also supports the role of RAS in partial adrenalectomy [161]. With robotic partial adrenalectomy, successful preservation of adrenocortical function is achieved [162].

RAS is an emerging technique for the treatment of pancreatic neoplasms. Robotic spleen-preserving distal pancreatectomy for a solid pseudopapillary tumor in pediatric patient, can be considered in younger patients presenting with a solid pseudopapillary tumor in the distal pancreas, and its use as an alternative to open pancreatectomy [163]. A report with 15 adolescents with pancreatic head tumor treated with MIS. Pancreaticoduodenectomy was performed, 10 cases with conventional laparoscopic surgery and 5 cases with RAS. The pathological diagnoses were solid pseudopapillary neoplasms (8), neuroendocrine neoplasms (3), intraductal papillary mucinous neoplasm (1), cystic fibroma (1), serous cystadenoma (1), Ewing's sarcoma (1). Six patients presented postoperative complications. The median follow-up was 37 months. The patient with Ewing's sarcoma was diagnosed with liver metastasis 41 months after surgery and died 63 months after surgery. All other patients survived without a tumor [164].

Robotic gynecological surgery in girls with ovarian disease, the ideal is to maintain the morphology of the ovary, which is beneficial for the recovery of postoperative ovarian function, especially in benign diseases. In centers where robotic surgery is available, ovarian tumors are a suitable entry procedure [128].

Robotic surgery can also be used in supportive care in pediatric oncology including placement of gastrostomy tubes and ovarian transposition [104].

The fundamental oncological principles of no tumor spillage and total resection of tumor margins can be adhered to by RAS; a specific concern being the lack of haptics having an impact on the surgeon's ability to differentiate cancerous from healthy tissue. However, it has been noted that the loss of tactile feedback is, very well compensated for by the excellent optical system [158]. Cancer patients are necessarily followed for recurrences, and only long-term prospective studies of robotic resections can guarantee adherence of the RAS to oncological principles.

Contraindications in children for MIS in tumors, including robotic surgery, are large or fragile tumors that carry a high risk of fracture and tumor spillage, significant adhesions from previous operations, and significant deterioration of respiratory or cardiovascular physiology [104].

## 7. Otorhinolaryngology

Pediatric robotic surgery has been used least frequently in otorhinolaryngology [72]. Until now, the majority of RAS applications in otorhinolaryngology is a transoral approach, particularly useful in masses of the base of the tongue. Open surgery can facilitate access to the oropharyngeal region, including the base of the tongue, but can lead to the morbidity of splitting the lip and jaw or require pharyngotomy. As a result, the robotic transoral approach is being used [165]. In the near future, we believe that transoral robotic surgery may become the gold standard.

In a publication of pediatric cases of robotic transoral surgery, with 41 patients, with age between 2 months and 19 years, the techniques were, lingual tonsillectomies (16), lingual and lingual based tonsillectomies (9), 2 malignant diseases in the oropharynx (high-grade undifferentiated sarcoma and biphasic synovial sarcoma), a thyroglossal duct cyst at the base of the tongue, laryngeal cleft cysts (11), a posterior glottic stenosis, and a surgery for congenital true vocal cord paralysis. A minor intraoperative complication occurred. No patient required postoperative tracheostomy. Conversion index was 9.8% [166].

## 8. Author's experience in robotic surgery

From March 2015 to January 2021, since the beginning the prospective registry of the casuistry has been carried out. We have performed 258 robot-assisted laparoscopic and thoracoscopic surgeries (RALTS) in 227 patients (224 children and 3 adults), in a public hospital and two private hospitals in Mexico City. The demographic data of the patients are, in relation to gender, 52.4% male and 47.6% female. The average and range of age, weight and height of the patients were, age 79.5 months (2 to 204), weight 26.8 kg (4.4 to 102) and height 114.5 cm (55 to 185), the smallest patient was 2 months old, 4.4 kg in weight and 57 cm in height, a left pyeloplasty was performed. The adult patients were 31, 63 and 64 years old.

We grouped our RALTS into gastrointestinal-hepatobiliary 123 (47.68%), urological 117 (45.35%), thoracic 10 (3.87% and oncological 8 (3.1%). We have performed 46 different techniques, globally our conversion rate is 3.1%, the hemotransfusion rate is 4.2%, the mean postoperative stay is 2.5 days, and the mean follow-up is 40 months.

From the group of gastrointestinal-hepatobiliary robotic surgery, in order of frequency, the techniques performed were: primary fundoplication 50 (41.67%), redo fundoplication 20 (15.83%), gastrostomy 17 (14.16%), cholecystectomy 14 (11.67%), biliodigestive 7 (5%), being 5 resections of choledochal cysts with hepaticojejunostomy, a Kasai operation and a hepaticojejunostomy to manage the lesion of the left hepatic duct. Splenectomy 6 (5%), Malone operation 2 (1.67%) and various techniques 7 (5%), of single cases, duodenoplasty and adhesiolysis, gastric trichobezoar extraction, drainage of recurrent retrohepatic abscess after appendectomy, gastric antrum membrane resection, gastrojejunostomy de-derivation, and Ladd's Cure. In this group of gastro-intestinal-hepatobiliary robotic surgery, the conversion rate was 3.25%, intraoperative complications 1.6%, and postoperative complications 4%. In this group of RAS 14 different techniques were performed.

From the robotic urological surgery group, in order of frequency, the techniques performed were: pyeloplasty 26 (22.2%), ureteral reimplantation 21 (17.94%), nephrectomy 20 (17.1%), Mitrofanoff operation 8 (6.8%), nephroureterectomy 7 (6%), ureterostomy de-derivation and ureteral neo-reimplantation 5 (4.3%), nephro-cystolithotomy 5 (4.3%), varicocelectomy 5 (4.3%), release of extrinsic UPJ obstruction 4 (3.4%), inguinal hernioplasty 3 (2.56%) and various techniques 13 (11.1%) of single cases, ureteroureterostomy, augmentation cystoplasty, bladder neck closure, heminephroureterectomy, perirenal abscess drainage, colostomy closure, enterovesical fistula closure, Mitrofanoff review, ureterostomy and ureteropyelography, bilateral gonadectomy, duplicated ureter ureterostomy, hysterosalpingectomy, bladder wall biopsy. In this robotic urologic surgery group, the conversion rate was 0.85%, intraoperative complications 0.85%, and postoperative complications 1.7%. In this group of RAS 20 different techniques were performed.

In the robotic thoracic surgery group, in order of frequency, the techniques performed were: lobectomy 4 (40%), diaphragmatic plication or plasty 4 (40%), a bronchogenic cyst resection (10%) and a pleural biopsies (10%). In this robotic thoracic surgery group, the conversion rate was 20% and postoperative complications 10%. In this group of RAS 5 different techniques were performed.

In the robotic oncological surgery group, the techniques performed were adrenalectomy 2 (for adenoma and another for pheochromocytoma) and single techniques of, anterior mediastinal teratoma resection, Ewing tumor resection, Wilms tumor stage 3 resection in horseshoe kidney, partial gastrectomy for carcinoid tumor, retroperitoneal lipoma resection and conservative resection of ovarian cyst. In this robotic cancer surgery group, the conversion rate was 12.5%, and there were no complications. In this group of RAS 8 different techniques were performed. The cases of adult patients were pheochromocytoma, adrenal adenoma and carcinoid tumor.

Previously, we published our experience with RALTS, the first 186 surgeries [14], the first 4 cases of choledochal cyst resection [109], redo Nissen fundoplication [114] and in thoracic surgery [133].

## 9. Implementation of a pediatric robotic surgery program

### 9.1 Planning

The success of a pediatric robotic surgery program (PRSP) depends on a well-structured plan. Implementing a PRSP requires institutional support and requires a comprehensive, detail-oriented plan that takes into account training, supervision, cost, and cases volume. Given the lower prevalence of robotic surgery in children, in many cases it may be more feasible to implement pediatric robotic surgery within an adult robotic surgery program. The pediatric surgery team determines its goals for volume expansion, surgical case selection, surgeons training, and surgical innovation within the specialty. In addition to the clinical model, a robust economic model that includes marketing must be present, especially in private hospitals [167].

### 9.2 Development of the program

The development of a robotic surgery program is associated with significant initial costs due to the initial investment in the robotic surgical system [168]. Adequate surgical volume is essential for both feasibility and ensuring adequate results for patients [64]. The surgeon should start with less complex index cases and gradually progress to more advanced reconstructive procedures with growing experience [61].

Less complex cases, such as a fundoplication, are excellent robotic training cases not only for surgeons and anesthesia personnel, but also for technical and nursing personnel assisting in the operating room [169].

Additionally, robotic cholecystectomy is a suitable procedure for first few surgeries when pediatric surgeons are beginning robotic surgery [125]. It is imperative to have a core group of specific personnel familiar with robotic procedures to increase efficiency. Adequate and systematic performance of the entire team in simple cases, then translates into better performance in more complex cases.

It is estimated that approximately 100 cases are required to obtain consistent results in pediatric robotic surgery cases by a surgical team [167]. The learning curve for each procedure varies, but is shorter than with laparoscopy, for example for robotic pyeloplasty there are 15 to 20 cases, to obtain similar results and surgical success [170]. Experience shows that in complex or reconstructive techniques, surgeons using the open approach switch to the robot-assisted approach, such as pyeloplasty, ureteral reimplantation, biliodigestive and pulmonary lobectomy, among others.

### 9.3 Robotic pediatric surgery team

There are three main actors involved in the implementation of a pediatric robotic surgery program: i. Surgeons and anesthetists, ii. Nurses and iii. Administration [168].

Successful robotic surgery is mentioned as requiring four elements, i. Good understanding of the surgical procedure, ii. Excellent surgical skills, iii. Frequent teamwork training, and iv. Trocar placement [171]. Adequate surgical volume is critical both for feasibility and to ensure good patient outcomes. Cases should be performed once a week to maintain surgical skill and advance to more advanced reconstructive procedures.

There has been a growing role for simulation and surgical training. Currently, the robotic surgery simulators available for training are the Mimic and da Vinci simulators. The simulators evaluate the skills in the different tasks that the surgeon performs. It is desirable that surgeons have previous experience in conventional laparo-thoracoscopy.

### 9.4 Training, accreditation and credentialing

Training and accreditation. In the present, the certification process to be a robotic surgeon depends on the manufacturer. Intuitive Surgical (Sunnyvale, CA,

USA), the manufacturers of the da Vinci Surgical System, have a separate training program that takes surgeons from console setup to the monitoring phase for initial cases with support from a proctor.

This process should be more structured and create a curriculum for robotic surgeons, this is essential for the training and objective evaluation of future robotic surgeons. Defining results, specific training tasks and their validation; as well as, establishment of measurements and approval criteria to improve the quality of robotic surgery should be included in the plan [172]. Academic organizations and hospital institutions can lead the implementation of a structured curriculum.

An accreditation proposal for the robotic surgeon is the following; After the intuitive surgery training program (step 1), then do the first five cases with a co-surgeon (step 2), who has the dual role of preceptor and supervisor, assesses the surgeon who is learning and also imparts new skills and takes control of the operative case if the clinical situation warrants it (the tutor allows the trainee to gain robotic experience safely in the first index cases). This is followed by 6 to 10 cases in which the tutor / supervisor is a bedside assistant (step 3). The preceptor/supervisor reports the findings to the Institution's Robotics Committee on the skills and progress of the trainee, evaluating whether the independent practice can be continued by the surgeon (step 4), based on the favorable evaluation of the preceptor [167].

The author's experience supports this accreditation proposal so that the learning curve of the surgeon, who is starting his foray into robotic surgery, is a satisfactory experience for him, and the patient is offered the greatest security from the stage of the curve of learning.

### 9.5 Program information data log

Data collection is very important. Collecting, analyzing, and presenting data prospectively to Institutional colleagues, at a minimum, allow objective analysis of results for comparative studies against other approaches, as well as to publish them.

## 10. The future of robotic surgery in children

Recently, the Senhance Robotics System (Transenterix, Morrisville, NC) has begun offering 3 mm instrument sizes, which could make robotic surgery more technically feasible for even the smallest pediatric patient. Although not currently approved for use in pediatric surgery, the Transenterix platform, was evaluated in an experimental study where surgeons were able to successfully perform intracorporeal and knotted sutures in body cavities as small as 90 ml, and the instruments could be inserted directly without the need for ports, reducing the required distance between ports [5]. This Transenterix platform has haptic feedback.

With advancing technology and the demand for more compact robotic platforms, the future for robotic surgery will doubtlessly result in a reduction of instrument size and an improvement in haptic feedback. This puts the pediatric patient in particular, the newborn at the forefront. Reconstructive surgery such as esophageal and intestinal anastomosis, all of which require a delicate and more magnified approach will benefit enormously from these advances. The pediatric and neonatal patient must be at the forefront of research into the future of robotic surgery [173].

We are at a dawn of a new age in surgery, as we witness the dramatic growth in robotic surgery. The proliferation and commercialization of new robotic surgical systems over the next few years will drive competition, lower cost, and accelerate the adoption of these technologies [174].

Artificial intelligence. More sophisticated systems will track the surgeon's movements and patient data and synchronize with outcomes data to provide us with early warning systems for complications. One more interesting aspect is how these systems will participate in the surgical decision-making process in real time. We are already gathering data on tissue perfusion, helping us decide on the appropriate location for an anastomosis. Additionally, using artificial intelligence, real-time data will be collected from many sources, including electronic medical records, anesthesia monitoring systems, video images, and surgeon data for making decisions that we will increasingly rely on [174].

Digital surgery (Surgery 4.0), the next frontier of surgery, is defined as the convergence of surgical technology, real-time data and artificial intelligence. Following previous waves of disruption, which saw the transition from open (Surgery 1.0) to laparoscopic surgery (Surgery 2.0), and from laparoscopic surgery to robotic surgery (Surgery 3.0), the digital paradigm in surgery is bringing unprecedented changes to the century-old field. The power of linked data and advancements in artificial intelligence are beginning to make a real impact in the way surgeries are performed, reducing well-documented variability in surgical process and outcomes.

Companies, investors, surgeons and health systems are racing to accelerate the digitization of surgery in order to dramatically improve patient outcomes whilst reducing cost and inefficiencies; improve patient access; reduce inequities between populations; improve quality; and deliver more personalized surgical care, and the digital surgery is the next apex in surgery [175].

Verb Surgical is building a digital surgery platform that combines robotics, advanced visualization, advanced instrumentation, data analysis, and connectivity. Surgery 4.0 or digital, which seeks to achieve less invasive and smarter interventions, "marks the beginning of a true democratization of the discipline". The Verb Surgical platform will be an option in the near future of digital surgery [175, 176].

## 11. Conclusions

In this chapter, in relation to robot-assisted surgery, its definition, characteristics, advantages, benefits, limitations and applications in children are addressed. As well as, the surgical areas of its application in the pediatric population, which include urological, general, thoracic, oncological and otorhinolaryngological surgery.

To date, there are multiple publications that demonstrate that robotic surgery in children is safe and effective, and it is important to offer children its benefits. However, a frequent conclusion of published studies on robotic surgery in children is the impossibility of carrying out comparative studies with all the scientific rigor, which makes it impossible to reach solid conclusions about the advantages and benefits in the pediatric population.

Robotic surgery preferably applied to difficult and complex cases adds value to patient care, and is an important balancing factor against the apparently higher cost (main drawback), compared to open and laparo-thoracoscopic surgery.

The author included his results in pediatric robotic surgery, which compared to other series of similar published cases; the experience is favorable and encouraging.

Globally, to date, few pediatric surgeons have adopted the robot-assisted surgery, as opposed to more pediatric urologists who have benefited more children. To date, in malignant tumors in children, robotic surgery has been applied less.

Recommendations for the implementation of a pediatric robotic surgery program are included. With robotic assistance, it is important to mention that the learning curve is shorter than with laparo-thoracoscopic surgery. It is necessary for each institution to establish the curriculum for the accreditation and credentialing of the robotic surgeon. A proposal is included.

The future will be fascinating with upcoming advancements in robotic surgical systems, the use of artificial intelligence, and digital surgery.

## Acknowledgements

I thank the Pediatricians, Pediatric Surgery Residents and Pediatric Surgeons of the Department of Pediatrics of the Hospital Militar de Especialidades de la Mujer y Neonatología, for their collaboration in the referral of patients for treatment with robotic surgery, and your participation in the surgical teams or as trainees. As well as, the Pediatric Surgeons of the Hospital Angeles Lomas and the Hospital Español of Mexico City, who participated in the surgical teams as trainees.

## Conflict of interest

The author declares to be Proctor of the da Vinci Surgical System and sometimes receives salary for advice to Surgeons in their first robotic procedures. In relation to the execution of this manuscript, no economic financing was received.

## Author details

Mario Navarrete-Arellano
Hospital Central Militar and Hospital Angeles Lomas, Mexico City, Mexico

*Address all correspondence to: drcirugiaroboticamx@gmail.com

## References


[1] Ure B. Enthusiasm, evidence and ethics: the triple E of minimally invasive pediatric surgery. J Pediatr Surg. 2013;48(1):27-33. Doi: 10.1016/j.jpedsurg.2012.10.013

[2] Passerotti C, Peters CA. Pediatric robotic–assisted laparoscopy: adescription of the principle procedures. Sci World J. 2006;6:2581-2588. Doi: 10.1100/tsw.2006.399

[3] Fernandez N, Farhat WA. A comprehensive analysis of robot-assisted surgery uptake in the pediatric surgical discipline. Front Surg. 2019;12;6:9. Doi: 10.3389/fsurg.2019.00009

[4] Bruns NE, Soldes OS, Ponsky TA. Robotic surgery may not "make the cut" in pediatrics. Front Pediatr. 2015;12;3:10. Doi: 10.3389/fped.2015.00010

[5] Bergholz R, Botden S, Verweij J, Tytgat S, Van Gemert W, Boettcher M, et al. Evaluation of a new robotic-assisted laparoscopic surgical system for procedures in small cavities. J Robot Surg. 2020;14(1):191-197. Doi: 10.1007/s11701-019-00961-y

[6] Cundy TP, Harley SJD, Marcus HJ, Hughes-Hallett A, Khurana S. Global trends in paediatric robot assisted urological surgery: a bibliometric and Progressive Scholarly Acceptance analysis. J Robot Surg. 2018;12(1):109-15. Doi: 10.1007/s11701-017-0703-3

[7] Meininger D, Byhahn C, Markus BH, Heller K, Westphal K. Total endoscopic Nissen fundoplication with the robotic device "da Vinci" in children. Hemodynamics, gas exchange, and anesthetic management. Anaesthesist. 2001;50(4):271-275. Doi: 10.1007/s001010051001

[8] Gutt CN, Markus B, Kim ZG, Meininger D, Brinkmann L, Heller K. Early experiences of robotic surgery in children. Surg Endosc. 2002;16(7):1083-1086. Doi: 10.1007/s00464-001-9151-1

[9] Heller K, Gutt C, Schaeff B, Beyer PA, Markus B. Use of the robot system Da Vinci for laparoscopic repair of gastro-oesophageal reflux in children. Eur J Pediatr Surg. 2002;12(4):239-242. Doi: 10.1055/s-2002-34489

[10] Meininger DD, Byhahn C, Heller K, Gutt CN, Westphal K. Totally endoscopic Nissen fundoplication with a robotic system in a child. Surg Endosc. 2001;15(11):1360. Doi: 10.1007/s00464-001-4200-3

[11] Lee RS, Retik AB, Borer JG, Peters CA. Pediatric robot assisted laparoscopic dismembered pyeloplasty: comparison with a cohort of open surgery. J Urol. 2006;175(2):683-687. Doi: 10.1016/S0022-5347(05)00183-7

[12] Peters CA. Robotically assisted surgery in pediatric urology. Urol Clin North Am. 2004;31(4):743-752. Doi: 10.1016/j.ucl.2004.06.007

[13] Cundy TP, Shetty K, Clark J, Chang TP, Sriskandarajah K, Gattas NE, et al. The first decade of robotic surgery in children. J Pediatr Surg. 2013; 48:858-865. Doi: 10.1016/j.jpedsurg.2013.01.031

[14] Navarrete-Arellano M, Garibay González F. Robot-Assisted Laparoscopic and Thoracoscopic Surgery: Prospective Series of 186 Pediatric Surgeries. Front Pediat. 2019;7:200. Doi: 10.3389/fped.2019.00200

[15] Meehan JJ. Robotic Surgery in Small Children: Is There Room for This? J Laparoendosc Adv Surg Tech A. 2009;19(5):707-12. Doi: 10.1089/lap.2008.0178

[16] Barkun JS, Aronson JK, Feldman LS, Maddern GJ, Strasberg SM, Balliol

Collaboration, et al. Evaluation and stages of surgical innovations. Lancet. 2009;374(9695):1089-1096. Doi: 10.1016/S0140-6736(09)61083-7

[17] Bax NMA. Karl Storz Lecture. Ten years of maturation of endoscopic surgery in children. Is the wine good? J Pediatr Surg. 2004;39(2):146-151. Doi: 10.1016/j.jpedsurg.2003.10.016

[18] Wilson CB. Adoption of new surgical technology. BMJ 2006;332(7553):112-114. Doi: 10.1136/bmj.332.7533.112

[19] Mirheydar HS, Parsons JK. Diffusion of robotics into clinical practice in the United States: process, patient safety, learning curves, and the public health. World J Urol. 2013; 31(3):455-461. Doi: 10.1007/s00345-012-1015-x

[20] Meehan JJ, Sandler A. Robotic surgery: a single- institutional review of the first 100 consecutive cases. Surg Endosc. 2008;22:177-182. Doi: 10.1007/s00464-007-9418-2

[21] de Lamberg G, Fourcade L, Centi J, Fredon F, Braik K, Szwarc C, et al. How to successfully implement a robotic pediatric surgery program: lessons learned after 96 procedures. Surg Endosc. 2013;27:2137-2144. Doi: 10.1007/s00464-012-2729-y

[22] Sinha SK, Haddad M. Robot-assisted surgery in children: current status. J Robotic Surg. 2008;1:243-246. Doi: 10.1007/s11701-007-0054-6

[23] Alqahtani A, Albassam A, Zamakhshary M, Shoukri M, Altokhais T, Aljazairi A, et al. Robot-assisted pediatric surgery: how far can we go? World J Surg. 2010;34:975-978. Doi: 10.1007/s00268-010-0431-6

[24] Al-Bassam A. Robotic-assisted surgery in children: advantages and limitations. J Robot Surg. 2010;4:19-22. Doi: 10.1007/s11701-010-0181-3

[25] Camps JI. The use of robotics in pediatric surgery: my initial experience. Pediatr Surg Int. 2011;27:991-996. Doi: 10.1007/s00383-011-2901-9

[26] Marhuenda C, Giné C, Asensio M, Guillén G, Martínez Ibáñez V. Robotic surgery: first pediatric series in Spain. Cir Pediatr. 2011;24:90-92.

[27] Ballouhey Q, Villemagne T, Cros J, Szwarc C, Braik K, Longis B, et al. A comparison of robotic surgery in children weighing above and below 15.0 kg: size does not affect surgery success. Surg Endosc. 2015;29:2643-50. Doi: 10.1007/s00464-014-3982-z

[28] Bütter A, Merritt N, Dave S. Establishing a pediatric robotic surgery program in Canada. J Robot Surg. 2017;11:207-10. Doi: 10.1007/s11701-016-0646-0

[29] Mattioli G, Pini Prato A, Razore B, Leonelli L, Pio L, Avanzini S, et al. Da Vinci robotic surgery in a pediatric hospital. J Laparoendosc Adv Surg Tech A. 2017;27:539-45. Doi: 10.1089/lap.2016.0390

[30] Passerotti CC, Nguyen HT, Eisner BH, Lee RS, Peters CA. Laparoscopic reoperative pediatric pyeloplasty with robotic assistance. J Endourol. 2007;21:1137-40. Doi: 10.1089/end.2007.9929

[31] Volfson IA, Munver R, Esposito M, Dakwar G, Hanna M, Stock JA. Robot-assisted urologic surgery: safety and feasibility in the pediatric population. J Endourol. 2007;21:1315-8. Doi: 10.1089/end.2007.9982

[32] Lee RS, Passerotti CC, Cendron M, Estrada CR, Borer JG, Peters CA. Early results of robot assisted laparoscopic lithotomy in adolescents. J Urol.

2007;177:2306-10. Doi: 10.1016/j.juro.2007.01.178

[33] Franco I, Dyer LL, Zelkovic P. Laparoscopic pyeloplasty in the pediatric patient: hand sewn anastomosis versus robotic assisted anastomosis: is there a difference? J Urol. 2007;178:1483-6. Doi: 10.1016/j.juro.2007.06.012

[34] Yee DS, Shanberg AM, Duel BP, Rodriguez E, Eichel L, Rajpoot D. Initial comparison of robotic-assisted laparoscopic versus open pyeloplasty in children. Urology. 2006;67:599-602. Doi: 10.1016/j.urology.2005.09.021

[35] Casale P. Robotic pediatric urology. Curr Urol Rep. 2009;10:115-8. Doi: 10.1007/s11934-009-0021-z

[36] Christman MS, Casale P. Robot-assisted bladder diverticulectomy in the pediatric population. J Endourol. 2012;26:1296-300. Doi: 10.1089/end.2012.0051

[37] Bansal D, Cost NG, Bean CM, Riachy E, Defoor WR Jr, Reddy PP, et al. Comparison of pediatric robotic-assisted laparoscopic nephroureterectomy and laparoendoscopic single-site nephroureterectomy. Urology. 2014; 83:438-42. Doi: 10.1016/j.urology.2013.08.066

[38] Mason MD, Anthony Herndon CD, Smith-Harrison LI, Peters CA, Corbett ST. Robotic-assisted partial nephrectomy in duplicated collecting systems in the pediatric population: techniques and outcomes. J Pediatr Urol. 2014;10:374-9. Doi: 10.1016/j.jpurol.2013.10.014

[39] Liu DB, Ellimoottil C, Flum AS, Casey JT, Gong EM. Contemporary national comparison of open, laparoscopic, and robotic-assisted laparoscopic pediatric pyeloplasty. J Pediatr Urol. 2014;10:610-5. Doi: 10.1016/j.jpurol.2014.06.010

[40] Esposito C, Masieri L, Steyaert H, Escolino M, Cerchione R, La Manna A, et al. Robot-assisted extravesical ureteral reimplantation (REVUR) for unilateral vesico-ureteral reflux in children: results of a multicentric international survey.World J Urol. 2018;36:481-8. Doi: 10.1007/s00345-017-2155-9

[41] Kawal T, Srinivasan AK, Chang J, Long C, Chu D, Shukla AR. Robotic assisted laparoscopic ureteral re-implant (RALUR): can post-operative urinary retention be predicted? J Pediatr Urol. 2018;14:323.e1-5. Doi: 10.1016/j.jpurol.2018.05.010

[42] Varda BK, Wang Y, Chung BI, Lee RS, Kurtz MP, Nelson CP. Has the robot caught up? National trends in utilization, perioperative outcomes, and cost for open, laparoscopic, and robotic pediatric pyeloplasty in the United States from 2003 to 2015. J Pediatr Urol. 2018;14:336.e1-8. Doi: 10.1016/j.jpurol.2017.12.010

[43] Monn MF, Bahler CD, Schneider EB, Whittam BM, Misseri R, Rink RC, et al. Trends in robot-assisted laparoscopic pyeloplasty in pediatric patients. Urology. 2013;81:1336-41. Doi: 10.1016/j.urology.2013.01.025

[44] Sukumar S, Roghmann F, Sood A, Abdo A, Menon M, Sammon JD, et al. Correction of ureteropelvic junction obstruction in children: national trends and comparative effectiveness in operative outcomes. J Endourol. 2014;28:592-8. Doi: 10.1089/end.2013.0618

[45] Varda BK, Johnson EK, Clark C, Chung BI, Nelson CP, Chang SL. National trends of perioperative outcomes and costs for open, laparoscopic and robotic pediatric pyeloplasty. J Urol. 2014;191:1090-5. Doi: 10.1016/j.juro.2013.10.077

[46] Garcia I, Salas de Armas IA, Pimpalwar A. Current trends in pediatric robotic surgery. Bangladesh J Endosurg. 2014;2:15-28. Doi: 10.3329/bje.v2i1.19589

[47] van Haasteren G, Levine S, Hayes W. Pediatric robotic surgery: early assessment. Pediatrics. 2009;124(6):1642-1649. Doi: 10.1542/peds.2008-3822

[48] Villanueva J, Killian M, Chaudhry R. Robotic urologic surgery in the infant: a review. Curr Urol Rep. 2019;18;20(7):35. Doi: 10.1007/s11934-019-0902-8

[49] Najmaldin A, Antao B. Early experience of tele-robotic sugery in children. Int J Med Robot Comp Assist Surg. 2007;3:199-202. Doi: 10.1002/rcs.150

[50] Gattas N, Smith C, Alizai NK, Wyk V, Sellors J, Whiteley S, et al. Short and long term complications of robotic abdominal surgery in children. In: Presented at the 5th Hamlyn Symposium on Medical Robotics, London, United Kingdom, July 1-2, 2012; 11. Avaliable online at: http://ubimon.doc.ic.ac.uk/Hamlyn2012/public/Hamlyn_2012_proceedings_2.pdf

[51] Bansal D, Defoor WR Jr, Reddy PP, Minevich EA, Noh PH. Complications of robotic surgery in pediatric urology: a single institution experience. Urology. 2013;82:917-20. Doi: 10.1016/j.urology.2013.05.046

[52] The dictionary by Farlex, Segen Medical Dictionary [Internet]. 2020. Available from: https://medicaldictionary.thefreedictionary.com/robotic+surgery [Accedded: 2020-12-14]

[53] Medical Advisory Secretariat. Robotic-assisted minimally invasive surgery for gynecologic and urologic oncology: an evidence-based analysis. Ont Health Technol Assess Ser 2010;10:1-118.

[54] Westebring-van der Putten EP, Goossens RHM, Jakimowicz JJ, Dankelman J. Haptics in minimally invasive surgery—a review. Minimally Invas Ther. 2008; 17:3-16. Doi: 10.1080/13645700701820242

[55] Braumann C, Jacobi CA, Menenakos C, Ismail M, Rueckert JC, Mueller JM. Robotic-assisted laparoscopic and thoracoscopic surgery with the da Vinci system: a 4-year experience in a single institution. Surg Laparosc Endosc Percutan Tech. 2008;18:260-266. Doi: 10.1097/SLE.0b013e31816f85e5

[56] Vereczkel A, Bubb H, Feussner H. Laparoscopic surgery and ergonomics: it's time to think of ourselves as well. Surg Endosc. 2003;17:1680-1682. Doi: 10.1007/s00464-003-9020-1

[57] Lee H, Hirose S, Bratton B, Farmer D. Initial experience with complex laparoscopic biliary surgery in children: biliary atresia and choledochal cyst. J Pediatr Surg. 2004;39(6):804-807. Doi: 10.1016/j.jpedsurg.2004.02.018

[58] Qu X, Cui L, Xu J. Laparoscopic Surgery in the treatment of children with Choledochal Cyst. Pak J Med Sci. 2019;35(3):807-811. Doi: 10.12669/pjms.35.3.85

[59] Lee JR. Anesthetic considerations for robotic surgery. Korean J Anesthesiol. 2014;66(1):3-11. Doi: 10.4097/kjae.2014.66.1.3

[60] Munoz CJ, Nguyen HT, Houck CS. Robotic surgery and anesthesia for pediatric urologic procedures. Curr Opin Anaesthesiol. 2016;29(3):337-44. Doi: 10.1097/ACO.0000000000000333

[61] Herron DM, Marohn M. A Consensus Document on Robotic Surgery. SAGES [Internet]. 2007.

Avaliable from: https://www.sages.org/publications/guidelines/consensus-document-robotic-surgery/ [Accessed: 2020-12-14]

[62] Childers CP, Maggard-Gibbons M. Estimation of the acquisition and operating costs for robotic surgery. JAMA. 2018;320(8):835-836. Doi: 10.1001/jama.2018.9219

[63] O'Kelly F, Farhat WA, Koyle MA. Cost, training and simulation models for robotic assisted surgery in pediatric urology. World J Urol. 2020;38(8):1875-1882. Doi: 10.1007/s00345-019-02822-7

[64] Palmer KJ, Lowe GJ, Coughlin GD, Patil N, Patel VR. Launching a successful robotic surgery program. J Endourol. 2008;22(4):819-24. Doi: 10.1089/end.2007.9824

[65] Baek SK, Carmichael JC, Pigazzi A. Robotic surgery: colon and rectum. Cancer J. 2013;19(2):140-6. Doi: 10.1097/PPO.0b013e31828ba0fd

[66] Debernardo R, Starks D, Barker N, Armstrong A, Kunos CA. Robotic surgery in gynecologic oncology. Obstet Gynecol Int. 2011;2011:139867. Doi: 10.1155/2011/139867

[67] Buchs NC, Pugin F, Chassot G, Volonte F, Koutny-Fong P, Hagen ME, et al. Robot-assisted Roux-en-Y gastric bypass for super obese patients: a comparative study. Obes Surg. 2013;23(3):353-7. Doi: 10.1007/s11695-012-0824-8

[68] Hagen ME, Pugin F, Chassot G, Huber O, Buchs N, Iranmanesh P, et al. Reducing cost of surgery by avoiding complications: the model of robotic Roux-en-Y gastric bypass. Obes Surg. 2012;22(1):52-61. Doi: 10.1007/s11695-011-0422-1

[69] Rowe CK, Pierce MW, Tecci KC, Houck CS, Mandell J, Retik AB, et al. A comparative direct cost analysis of pediatric urologic robot-assisted laparoscopic surgery versus open surgery: Could robot-assisted surgery be less expensive? J Endourol. 2012;26:871-877. Doi: 10.1089/end.2011.0584

[70] Behan JW, Kim SS, Dorey F, De Filippo RE, Chang AY, Hardy BE, et al. Human capital gains associated with robotic assisted laparoscopic pyeloplasty in children compared to open pyeloplasty. J Urol. 2011;186 (4 Suppl):1663-1667. Doi: 10.1016/j.juro.2011.04.019

[71] Chaussy Y, Becmeur F, Lardy H, Aubert D. Robot-assisted surgery: current status evaluation in abdominal and urological pediatric surgery. J Laparoendosc Adv Surg Tech. 2013;23:530-538. Doi: 10.1089/lap.2012.0192

[72] Mehta D, Duvvuri U. Robotic surgery in pediatric otolaryngology: emerging trends. Laryngoscope. 2012;122 Suppl 4:S105-S106. Doi: 10.1002/lary.23806

[73] Szavay PO. Applications of Laparoscopic Transperitoneal Surgery of the Pediatric Urinary Tract. Front. Pediatr.2019; 7:29. Doi: 10.3389/fped.2019.00029

[74] Blanc T, Pio L, Clermidi P, Muller C, Orbach D, Minard-Colin V, et al. Robotic-assisted laparoscopic management of renal tumors in children: Preliminary results. Pediatr Blood Cancer. 2019;66 Suppl 3:e27867. Doi: 10.1002/pbc.27867

[75] Lee RS, Sethi AS, Passerotti CC, Retik AB, Borer JG, Nguyen HT, et al. Robot assisted laparoscopic partial nephrectomy: A viable and safe option in children. J Urol. 2009;181(2):823-8. Discussion 828-829. Doi: 10.1016/j.juro.2008.10.073

[76] Morales-López RA, Pérez-Marchán M, Pérez Brayfield M. Current

concepts in pediatric robotic assisted pyeloplasty. Front Pediatr. 2019; 24;7:4. Doi: 10.3389/fped.2019.00004

[77] Chan YY, Durbin-Johnson B, Sturm RM, Kurzrock EA. Outcomes after pediatric open, laparoscopic, and robotic pyeloplasty at academic institutions. J Pediatr Urol. 2017;13:49. e1-6. Doi: 10.1016/j.jpurol.2016.08.029

[78] Song SH, Lee C, Jung J, Kim SJ, Park S, Park H, et al. Comparative study of pediatric open pyeloplasty, laparoscopy-assisted extracorporeal pyeloplasty, and robot-assisted laparoscopic pyeloplasty. PLoS ONE. 2017; 12:e0175026. Doi: 10.1371/journal.pone.0175026

[79] Neheman A, Kord E, Zisman A, Darawsha AE, Noh PH. Comparison of robotic pyeloplasty and standard laparoscopic pyeloplasty in infants: a bi-institutional study. J Laparoendosc Adv Surg Tech A. 2018;28:467-70. Doi: 10.1089/lap.2017.0262

[80] Howe A, Kozel Z, Palmer L. Robotic surgery in pediatric urology. Asian J Urol. 2017; 4:55-67. Doi: 10.1016/j.ajur.2016.06.002

[81] Avery DI, Herbst KW, Lendvay TS, Corbett ST, Peters CA, Kim C. Robot-assisted laparoscopic pyeloplasty: multi-institutional experience in infants. J Pediatr Urol. 2015;11(3):139.e1-5. Doi: 10.1016/j.jpurol.2014.11.025.

[82] Crisan N, Neiculescu C, Matei DV, Coman I. Robotic retroperitoneal approach - a new technique for the upper urinary tract and adrenal gland. Int J Med Robot. 2013;9(4):492-6. Doi: 10.1002/rcs.1523

[83] Lowe GJ, Canon SJ, Jayanthi VR. Laparoscopic reconstructive options for obstruction in children with duplex renal anomalies. BJU Int. 2008;101:227-230. Doi: 10.1111/j.1464-410X.2007.07106.x

[84] Smith KM, Shrivastava D, Ravish IR, Nerli RB, Shukla AR. Robot-assisted laparoscopic ureteroureterostomy for proximal ureteral obstructions in children. J Pediatr Urol. 2009;5:475-9. Doi: 10.1016/j.jpurol.2009.03.004

[85] Passerotti CC, Diamond DA, Borer JG, Eisner BH, Barrisford G, Nguyen HT. Robot-assisted laparoscopic ureteroureterostomy: Description of technique. J Endourol. 2008;22:581-584. Doi: 10.1089/end.2007.9838

[86] Casale P, Mucksavage P, Resnick M, Kim SS. Robotic ureterocalicostomy in the pediatric population. J Urol. 2008;180(6):2643-2648. Doi: 10.1016/j.juro.2008.08.052

[87] Ganpule AP, Sripathi V. How small is small enough? Role of robotics in paediatric urology. J Min Access Surg. 2015;11(1):45-49. Doi: 10.4103/0972-9941.147689

[88] Baek M, Koh CJ. Lessons learned over a decade of pediatric robotic ureteral reimplantation. Investig Clin Urol. 2017;58(1):3-11. Doi: 10.4111/icu.2017.58.1.3

[89] Sahadev R, Spencer K, Srinivasan AK, Long CJ and Shukla AR. The Robot-Assisted Extravesical Anti-reflux Surgery: How We Overcame the Learning Curve. Front. Pediatr. 2019;7:93. Doi: 10.3389/fped.2019.00093

[90] Streem SB, Franke JJ, Smith JA. Management of upper urinary tract obstruction. In: Walsh PC, Retik AB, Vaughan ED Jr, et al. editors. Campbell's urology. 8th edition. Philadelphia: W. B. Saunders Co, 2003:463-512.

[91] Farina A, Esposito C, Escolino M, Lopez M, Settimi A, Varlet F. Laparoscopic extravesical ureteral reimplantation (LEVUR): a systematic review. Transl Pediatr. 2016;5:291-294. Doi: 10.21037/tp.2016.10.01

[92] Boysen WR, Akhavan A, Ko J, Ellison JS, Lendvay TS, Huang J, et al. Prospective multicenter study on robot-assisted laparoscopic extravesical ureteral reimplantation (RALUR-EV): Outcomes and complications. J Pediatr Urol. 2018;14(3):262.e1-262.e6. Doi: 10.1016/j.jpurol.2018.01.020

[93] Mitrofanoff P. Trans-appendicular continent cystostomy in the management of the neurogenic bladder. Chir Pediatr. 1980;21:297-305.

[94] Rodriguez MV, Wallace A, Gundeti MS. Robotic Bladder Neck Reconstruction with Mitrofanoff Appendicovesicostomy in a Neurogenic Bladder Patient. Urology. 2020;137:206-207. Doi: 10.1016/j.urology.2019.11.023

[95] Orvieto MA, Gundeti MS. Complex robotic reconstructive surgical procedures in children with urologic abnormalities. Curr Opin Urol. 2011;21(4):314-321. Doi: 10.1097/MOU.0b013e3283476f23

[96] Gargollo P. A critical evaluation of the role of robotic-assisted surgery in complex pediatric urology cases. Ann Transl Med. 2019;7(Suppl 3):S141. Doi: 10.21037/atm.2019.06.21

[97] Gargollo PC, Granberg C, Gong E, Tu D, Whittam B, Dajusta D . Complex Robotic Lower Urinary Tract Surgery in Patients with History of Open Surgery. J Urol. 2019;201:162-8. Doi: https://doi.org/10.1016/j.juro.2018.06.017

[98] Gundeti MS, Acharya SS, Zagaja GP, Shalhav AL. Paediatric robotic-assisted laparoscopic augmentation ileocystoplasty and Mitrofanoff appendicovesicostomy (RALIMA): Feasibility of and initial experience with the University of Chicago technique. BJU Int. 2011;107:962-9. Doi: 10.1111/j.1464-410X.2010.09706.x

[99] Zaragoza-Torresa RI, Galarza-Floresa ME, Gómez-Castellanosa JC Barrera-de León JC. Cambios urodinámicos posteriores a cirugía de ampliación vesical por vejiga neurogénica en pacientes pediátricos con mielomeningocele. Cirugía y Cirujanos. 2016;84(2):115-120. Doi: http://dx.doi.org/10.1016/j.circir.2015.10.008

[100] Rivera M, Granberg CF, Tollefson MK. Robotic-assisted laparoscopic surgery of urachal anomalies: a single-center experience. J Laparoendosc Adv Surg Tech A. 2015;25(4):291-4. Doi: 10.1089/lap.2014.0551

[101] Alsowayan O, Almodhen F, Alshammari A. Minimally invasive surgical approach to treat posterior urethral diverticulum. Urol Ann. 2015;7(2):273-6. Doi: 10.4103/0974-7796.152950

[102] Lima M, Maffi M, Di Salvo N, Ruggeri G, Libri M, Gargano T, et al. Robotic removal of Müllerian duct remnants in pediatric patients: our experience and a review of the literature. Pediatr Med Chir. 2018;30:40(1). Doi: 10.4081/pmc.2018.182

[103] Hidalgo-Tamola J, Sorensen MD, Bice JB, Lendvay TS. Pediatric robot-assisted laparoscopic varicocelectomy. J Endourol. 2009;23(8):1,297-1,300. Doi: 10.1089/end.2008.0523

[104] Petralia P. Pediatric robotic surgery. In: Mattioli G, Petralia P, editors. Pediatric Robotic Surgery. 1st ed. Cham, Switzerland: Springer International Publishing; 2017. p. 1-188

[105] Prato AP, Arnoldi R, Dusio MP, Cimorelli A, Barbetta V. Totally robotic soave pull-through procedure for Hirschsprung's disease: lessons learned from 11 consecutive pediatric patients. Pediatr Surg Int. 2020;36(2):209-218. Doi: 10.1007/s00383-019-04593-z

[106] Bütter A, Jayaraman S, Schlachta C. Robotic duodenojejunostomy for superior mesenteric artery syndrome in a teenager. J Robotic Surg. 2010; 4:265-269. Doi: 10.1007/s11701-010-0215-x

[107] Meejan JJ. Robotic repair of congenital duodenal atresia: a case report. J Pediatr Surg. 2007 ;42(7):E31-3. Doi: 10.1016/j.jpedsurg.2007.05.004

[108] Meehan JJ, Elliott S, Sandler A. The robotic approach to complex hepatobiliary anomalies in children: preliminary report. J Pediatr Surg. 2007;42, 2110-2114. Doi:10.1016/j.jpedsurg.2007.08.040

[109] Navarrete-Arellano M. Experience in the Treatment of Choledochal Cyst with Robot-Assisted Surgery in Children: and "The Current State of Minimally Invasive Surgery in this Anomaly'". Acta Scientific Paediatrics. 2019;2(11):04-13. Doi: 10.31080/ASPE.2019.02.0159

[110] Chen DX, Wang SJ, Jiang YN, Yu MC, Fan JZ, Wang XQ. Robot-assisted gallbladder-preserving hepatectomy for treating S5 hepatoblastoma in a child: A case report and review of the literature. World J Clin Cases. 2019;7(7): 872-880. Doi: 10.12998/wjcc.v7.i7.872

[111] Hambraeus M, Arnbjörnsson E, Anderberg M. A literature review of the outcomes after robot-assisted laparoscopic and conventional laparoscopic Nissen fundoplication for gastro-esophageal reflux disease in children. Int J Med Robot. 2013;9(4):428-32. Doi: 10.1002/rcs.1517

[112] Kang Y, Chen X, Wang B, Wang Z. Whether robot-assisted laparoscopic fundoplication is better for gastroesophageal reflux disease in adults: a systematic review and meta-analysis. Surg Endosc. 2010;24(8):1803-14. Doi: 10.1007/s00464-009-0873-9

[113] Sgarburã O, Tomulescu V, Blajut C, Popescu I. A 5-Year Perspective over Robotic General Surgery: Indications, Risk Factors and Learning Curves. Chirurgia. 2013;108(5): 599-610.

[114] Navarrete-Arellano M. Robotic-Assisted Laparoscopic Redo Nissen Fundoplication. Does it Offer Advantages in Children? Acad J Ped Neonatol. 2019;7(5):555781. Doi: 10.19080/AJPN.2019.07.555781

[115] Liem NT, Pham HD, Dung LA, Son TN, Vu HM. Early and intermediate outcomes of laparoscopic surgery for choledochal cysts with 400 patients. J Laparoendosc Adv Surg Tech A. 2012; 22(6): 599-603. Doi: 10.1089/lap.2012.0018

[116] Woo R, Le D, Albanese CT, Kim SS. Robot-assisted laparoscopic resection of a type I choledochal cyst in a child. J Laparoendosc Adv Surg Tech. 2006;16(2):179-83. Doi: 10.1089/lap.2006.16.179

[117] Chi SQ, Cao GQ, Li S, Guo JL, Zhang X, Ying Zhou Y, et al. Outcomes in robotic versus laparoscopic-assisted choledochal cyst excision and hepaticojejunostomy in children. Surg Endosc. 2020. Doi: 10.1007/s00464-020-07981-y

[118] Dutta S, Woo R, Albanese CT. Minimal access portoenterostomy: Advantages and disadvantages of standard laparoscopic and robotic techniques. J Laparoendosc Adv Surg Tech A. 2007;17:258-264. Doi: 10.1089/lap.2006.0112

[119] Hu MG, Xiao YH, Song DD, Zhao GD, Liu YZ, Wang Z, Li HY, Liu R. First experience of robotic spleen-preserving distal pancreatectomy in a child with insulinoma. World J Surg Oncol. 2017;15(1):199. Doi: 10.1186/s12957-017-1265-6

[120] Tian F, Hong XF, Wu WM, Han XL, Wang MY, Cong L, et al.

Propensity score-matched analysis of robotic versus open surgical enucleation for small pancreatic neuroendocrine tumours. Br J Surg. 2016;103(10):1358-1364. Doi: 10.1002/bjs.10220

[121] Liang M, Jiang J, Dai H, Hong X, Han X, Cong L, et al. Robotic enucleation for pediatric insulinoma with MEN1 syndrome: a case report and literature review. BMC Surgery. 2018;18(1):44. Doi: 10.1186/s12893-018-0376-5

[122] Hebra A, Smith VA, Lesher AP. Robotic Swenson pull-through for Hirschsprung's disease in infants. Am Surg. 2011;77(7):937-941. Doi: 10.1308/rcsann.supp2.18

[123] Raissi B, Taylor BM, Taves DH. Recurrent superior mesenteric artery (Wilkie's) syndrome: a case report. Can J Surg. 1996;39(5):410-416.

[124] Ayloo SM, Masrur MA, Bianco FM, Giulianotti PC. Robotic Roux-en-Y duodenojejunostomy for superior mesenteric artery syndrome: operative technique. J Laparoendosc Adv Surg Tech A. 2011;21(9):841-4. Doi: 10.1089/lap.2011.0070

[125] Ahn N, Signor G, Singh TP, Stain S, Whyte Ch. Robotic Single- and Multisite Cholecystectomy in Children. J Laparoendosc Adv Surg Tech A. 2015;25(12):1033-5. Doi: 10.1089/lap.2015.0106

[126] Shelby R, Kulaylat AN, Villella A, Michalsky MP, Diefenbach KA, Aldrink JH. A comparison of robotic-assisted splenectomy and laparoscopic splenectomy for children with hematologic disorders. J Pediatr Surg. 2020;S0022-3468(20)30615-1. Doi: 10.1016/j.jpedsurg.2020.08.031

[127] Nakib G, Calcaterra V, Scorletti F, Romano P, Goruppi I, Mencherini S, et al. Robotic assisted surgery in pediatric gynecology: promising innovation in mini invasive surgical procedures. J Pediatr Adolesc Gynecol. 2013;26(1): e5-7. Doi: 10.1016/j.jpag.2012.09.009

[128] Xie XX, Wang N, Wang ZH, Zhu YY, Wang JR, Wang XQ. Robotic-assisted resection of ovarian tumors in children: A case report and review of literature. World J Clin Cases. 2019;7(17):2542-2548. Doi: 10.12998/wjcc.v7.i17.2542

[129] Chaer RA, Jacobsen G, Elli F, Harris J, Goldstein A, Horgan S. Robotic-assisted laparoscopic pediatric Heller's cardiomyotomy: initial case report. J Laparoendosc Adv Surg Tech A. 2004;14(5):270-3. Doi: 10.1089/lap.2004.14.270

[130] Altokhais T, Mandora H, Al-Qahtani A, Al-Bassam A. Robot-assisted Heller's myotomy for achalasia in children. Comput Assist Surg. 2016; 21(1): 127-131. Doi: 10.1080/24699322.2016.1217352

[131] Galvani C, Gorodner MV, Moser F, Baptista M, Donahue P, Horgan S. Laparoscopic Heller myotomy for achalasia facilitated by robotic assistance. Surg Endosc. 2006;20:1105-1112. Doi: 10.1007/s00464-005-0272-9

[132] Rodríguez RM, Kalfa N, Allal H. Advantages of robot-assisted surgery in anorectal malformations: Report of a case. J Minim Access Surg. 2016;12(2):176-8. Doi: 10.4103/0972-9941.169988

[133] Navarrete-Arellano M. Thoracic surgery by minimally invasion robot-assisted in children: "experience and current status". Mini-invasive Surg. 2020;4:9. Doi: 10.20517/2574-1225.2019.70

[134] Le Bret E, Papadatos S, Folliguet T, Carbognani D, Pétrie J, Aggoun Y, et al. Interruption of patent ductus arteriosus in childre: Robotically assisted versus

videothoracoscopic surgery. J Thorac Cardiovasc Surg. 2002;123:973-6. Doi: 10.1067/mtc.2002.121049

[135] Mihaljevic T, Cannon JW, del Nido PJ. Robotically assisted division of a vascular ring in children. J Thorac Cardiovasc Surg. 2003;125:1163-4. Doi: 10.1067/mtc.2003.52

[136] Ballouhey Q, Villemagne T, Cros J, Virginie Vacquerie V, Bérenguer D, Karim Braik K, et al. Assessment of paediatric thoracic robotic surgery. Interactive Cardiovascular and Thoracic Surgery. 2015; 20(3): 300-303. Doi: 10.1093/icvts/ivu406

[137] Park BJ, Flores RM, Rusch VW. Robotic assistance for video-assisted thoracic surgical lobectomy: technique and initial results. J Thorac Cardiovasc Surg. 2006;131:54-9. Doi: 10.1016/j.jtcvs.2005.07.031

[138] Wei S, Chen M, Chen N, Liu L. Feasibility and safety of robot-assisted thoracic surgery for lung lobectomy in patients with non-small cell lung cancer: a systematic review and meta-analysis. World J Surg Oncol. 2017;15(1):98. Doi: 10.1186/s12957-017-1168-6

[139] Slater BJ, Meehan JJ. Robotic repair of congenital diaphragmatic anomalies. J Laparoendosc Adv Surg Tech A. 2009;19 Suppl 1:S123-7. Doi: 10.1089/lap.2008.0200.supp

[140] Rückert JC, Swierzy M, Ismail M. Comparison of robotic and nonrobotic thoracoscopic thymectomy: a cohort study. J Thorac Cardiovasc Surg. 2011;141:673-7. Doi: 10.1016/j.jtcvs.2010.11.042

[141] Rodriguez M, Gomez MR, Howard FM, Taylor WF. Myasthenia gravis in children: long-term follow-up. Ann Neurol. 1983;13:504-10. Doi: 10.1002/ana.410130506

[142] Castro D, Derisavifard S, Anderson M, Greene M, Iannaccone S. Juvenile myasthenia gravis: a twenty-year experience. J Clin Neuromuscul Dis. 2013;14:95-102. Doi: 10.1097/CND.0b013e318253a48e

[143] Goldstein SD, Culbertson NT, Garrett D, Salazar JH, Arendonk KV, Kimberly McIltrot K, et al. Thymectomy for myasthenia gravis in children: a comparison of open and thoracoscopic approaches. J Pediatr Surg. 2015;50(01):92-97. Doi: 10.1016/j.jpedsurg.2014.10.005

[144] Ashfaq A, Bernes SM, Weidler EM, Notrica DM. Outcomes of thoracoscopic thymectomy in patients with juvenile myasthenia gravis. J Pediatr Surg. 2016;51(07):1078-1083. Doi: 10.1016/j.jpedsurg.2015.12.016

[145] Hartwich J, Tyagi S, Margaron F, Oitcica C, Teasley J, Lanning D. Robot-assisted thoracoscopic thymectomy for treating myasthenia gravis in children. J Laparoendosc Adv Surg Tech A. 2012;22(09):925-929. Doi: 10.1089/lap.2012.0042

[146] Marina AD, Kölbel H, Müllers M, Kaiser O, Ismail M, Swierzy M, et al. Outcome after Robotic-Assisted Thymectomy in Children and Adolescents with Acetylcholine Receptor Antibody-Positive Juvenile Myasthenia Gravis. Neuropediatrics. 2017;48(4):315-322. Doi: 10.1055/s-0037-1603775

[147] Kamran A, Hamilton TE, Zendejas B, Nath B, Jennings RW, Smithers CJ. Minimally invasive surgical approach for posterior tracheopexy to treat severe tracheomalacia: lessons learned from initial case series. J Laparoendosc Adv Surg Tech A. 2018;28:1525-30. Doi: 10.1089/lap.2018.0198

[148] Toker A, Ayalp K, Grusina-Ujumaza J, Kaba E. Resection of a bronchogenic cyst in the first decade of life with robotic surgery. Interact

Cardiovasc Thorac Surg. 2014;19:321-3. Doi: 10.1093/icvts/ivu113

[149] Asaf BB, Kumar A, Vijay CL. Robotic excision of paraesophageal bronchogenic cyst in a 9-year-old child. J Indian Assoc Pediatr Surg. 2015;20:191-3. Doi: 10.4103/0971-9261.164256

[150] van Dalen EC, de Lijster MS, Leijssen LGJ, Michiels EMC, Kremer LCM, Caron HN, et al. Minimally invasive surgery versus open surgery for the treatment of solid abdominal and thoracic neoplasms in children (Review). Cochrane Database Syst Rev. 2015;1(1):CD008403. Doi: 10.1002/14651858.CD008403.pub3

[151] Cundy TP, Marcus HJ, Clark J, Hughes-Hallett A, Mayer EK, Najmaldin AS, et al. Robot-assisted minimally invasive surgery for pediatric solid tumors: a systematic review of feasibility and current status. Eur J Pediatr Surg. 2014;24(2):127-35. Doi: 10.1055/s-0033-1347297

[152] Hassan M, Smith JM. Robotic assisted excision of a left ventricular myxoma. Interactive Cardiovascular and Thoracic Surgery. 2012;14(1): 113-114. Doi: 10.1093/icvts/ivr021

[153] DeUgarte DA, Teitelbaum D, Hirschl RB, Geiger JD. Robotic extirpation of complex massive esophageal leiomyoma. J Laparoendosc Adv Surg Tech A. 2008;18(2): 286-289. Doi: 10.1089/lap.2007.0067

[154] Meehan JJ, Sandler AD. Robotic resection of mediastinal masses in children. J Laparoendosc Adv Surg Tech A. 2008; 18(1):114-119. Doi: 10.1089/lap.2007.0092

[155] Chen DX, Hou YH, Jiang YN, Shao LW, Wang SJ, Wang XQ. Removal of pediatric stage IV neuroblastoma by robot-assisted laparoscopy: A case report and literature review. World J Clin Cases. 2019; 7(12): 1499-1507. Doi: 10.12998/wjcc.v7.i12.1499

[156] Uwaydah NI, Jones A, Elkaissi M, Yu Z, Palmer BW. Pediatric robot-assisted laparoscopic radical adrenalectomy and lymph-node dissection for neuroblastoma in a 15-month-old. J Robot Surg. 2014;8(3):289-93. Doi: 10.1007/s11701-013-0441-0

[157] Akar ME, Leezer KH, Yalcinkaya TM. Robot-assisted laparoscopic management of a case with juvenile cystic adenomyoma. Fertility and Sterility. 2010; 94(3): E55–E6. Doi: 10.1016/j.fertnstert.2010.06.001

[158] Anderberg M, Backman T, Annerstedt M. Robot-assisted radical cystoprostatectomy in a small child with rhabdomyosarcoma: a case report. J Robotic Surg. 2008;2:101-103. Doi: 10.1007/s11701-008-0089-3

[159] Cost NG, DaJusta DG, Granberg CF, Cooksey RM, Laborde CE, Wickiser JE, et al. Robot-assisted laparoscopic retroperitoneal lymph node dissection in an adolescent population. J Endourol. 2012;26(6):635-40. Doi: 10.1089/end.2011.0214

[160] Cost NG, Geller JI, DeFoor Jr WR, Wagner LM, Noh PH. A robotic-assisted laparoscopic approach for pediatric renal cell carcinoma allows for both nephron-sparing surgery and extended lymph node dissection. J Pediatr Surg. 2012;47(10):1946-50. Doi: 10.1016/j.jpedsurg.2012.08.017

[161] Ball MW, Allaf ME. Robot-assisted adrenalectomy (total, partial, & metastasectomy). Urol Clin North Am. 2014;41(4):539-47. Doi: 10.1016/j.ucl.2014.07.008

[162] Julien JS, Ball D, Schulick R. Robot-assisted cortical-sparing adrenalectomy in a patient with Von Hippel-Lindau disease and bilateral

pheochromocytomas separated by 9 years. J Laparoendosc Adv Surg Tech A. 2006;16(5):473-7. Doi: 10.1089/lap.2006.16.473

[163] Lalli R, Merritt N, Schlachta CM, Bütter A. Robotic-assisted, spleen-preserving distal pancreatectomy for a solid pseudopapillary tumour in a pediatric patient: a case report and review of the literature. J Robot Surg. 2019;13(2):325-329. Doi: 10.1007/s11701-018-0835-0

[164] Jin WW, Lu C, Mou YP, Wang YY, Zhu QC, Xia T. Early experience of minimal invasive surgery for adolescent with pancreatic head tumor: a report of 15 cases. Zhonghua Wai Ke Za Zhi. 2020;58(7):512-515. Doi: 10.3760/cma.j.cn112139-20200211-00077

[165] Kayhan FT, Yigider AP, Koc AK, Kaya KH, Erdim I. Treatment of tongue base masses in children by transoral robotic surgery. Eur Arch Otorhinolaryngol. 2017;274(9):3457-3463. Doi: 10.1007/s00405-017-4646-0

[166] Erkul E, Duvvuri U, Mehta D, Aydil U. Transoral robotic surgery for the pediatric head and neck surgeries. Eur Arch Otorhinolaryngol. 2017;274(3):1747-1750. Doi: 10.1007/s00405-016-4425-3

[167] Murthy PB, Schadler ED, Orvieto M, Zagaja G, Shalhav AL, Gundeti MS. Setting up a pediatric robotic urology program: A USA institution experience. Int J Urol. 2018;25(2):86-93. Doi: 10.1111/iju.13415

[168] de Lambert G, Fourcade L, Centi J, Fredon F, Braik K, Szwarc C, at al. How to successfully implement a robotic pediatric surgery program: lessons learned after 96 procedures. Surg Endosc. 2013;27(6):2137-44. Doi: 10.1007/s00464-012-2729-y

[169] Meehan JJ, Meehan TD, Sandler A. Robotic fundoplication in children: resident teaching and a single institutional review of our first 50 patients. J Pediatr Surg. 2007;42(12):2022-5. Doi: 10.1016/j.jpedsurg.2007.08.022

[170] Sorensen MD, Delostrinos C, Johnson MH, Grady RW, Lendvay TS. Comparison of the learning curve and outcomes of robotic assisted pediatric pyeloplasty. J Urol. 2011;185(6 Suppl):2517-2522. Doi: 10.1016/j.juro.2011.01.021

[171] Chang C, Steinberg Z, Shah A, Gundeti MS. Patient positioning and port placement for robot-assisted surgery. J Endourol. 2014;28:631-638. Doi: 10.1089/end.2013.0733

[172] Patel VP. A Decade of Robotic Surgery: Past, Present and Future. In: Yang GZ, Darzi A (Eds). The Hamlyn Symposium on Medical Robotics. Imperial College London, UK. 1-2 July 2012. Page 5-6. ISBN: 978-0-9563776-3-0.

[173] Cave J, Clarke S. Paediatric robotic surgery. Ann R Coll Surg Engl. 2018;100(Suppl 7):18-21. Doi: 10.1308/rcsann.supp2.18

[174] Teixeira J. One Hundred Years of Evolution in Surgery: From Asepsis to Artificial Intelligence. Surg Clin North Am. 2020;100(2):xv-xvi. Doi: 10.1016/j.suc.2020.01.001

[175] https://www.digital.health/digital-surgery

[176] https://www.tynmagazine.com/que-es-la-cirugia-digital/ (Date Nov, 20, 2019).

Chapter 4

# Robotic Surgery for the Thoracic and Vascular Surgeon

*Lawek Berzenji, Krishan Yogeswaran, Patrick Lauwers, Paul Van Schil and Jeroen M.H. Hendriks*

## Abstract

In the last two decades, robotic-assisted approaches have gained popularity as alternatives to conventional open and minimal-invasive surgery (MIS). The robotic approach combines the concepts of the traditional MIS with the latest technological advancements, enabling the surgeon to control the instrumentation using a robotic device connected to a remote console. With this approach, the surgeon obviates the known drawbacks of conventional MIS, such as the reduced in-depth perception and hand-eye coordination. Since its introduction, numerous robotic-assisted procedures have been developed and tested across nearly all surgical fields. Data from previous studies have shown that a great majority of these techniques are feasible and have favourable treatment outcomes. In the field of thoracic and vascular surgery, two disciplines often combined in Belgium, robotic approaches have been implemented in the treatment of a wide array of disorders including lung cancer, mediastinal tumours, thoracic outlet syndrome, diaphragmatic paralysis, sympathectomy, aortobifemoral bypass surgery and division of the arcuate ligament for median arcuate ligament syndrome (MALS). Despite this increasing popularity, there are still a number of controversies regarding robotic surgery. There are only limited data on the cost-effectiveness of robotic surgery and its objective proven benefit over conventional MIS. In this review, we summarise the latest data on robotic approaches for the most relevant thoracic and vascular disorders.

**Keywords:** Robotic surgery, Minimal-invasive surgery, Thoracic surgery, Vascular surgery, RATS, VATS, RAAS

## 1. Introduction

The advent of minimally invasive surgery (MIS) has clearly changed the landscape for surgical practice worldwide. By combining multiple technological developments such as high-definition cameras and surgical microinstruments, surgeons are able to perform more and more complex procedures through small incisions [1]. Since the introduction of MIS, safe and feasible laparoscopic and thoracoscopic surgical procedures have been developed for a large variety of operations. For the majority of these procedures, studies have shown that the minimal-invasive approach results in fewer complications, reduced hospital stays, and faster return to normal functions compared to their respective open approach [2, 3]. However, despite these clear advantages of MIS, there are a number of drawbacks as well. Proficiency in MIS requires intensive, continuous training and often involves steep learning curves for surgeons in training. Despite their training, the surgeons are often confronted with a number of drawbacks such as poor depth perception, reduced spatial coordination due to the two-dimensional optics, a lack of instrument flexibility, reduced force feedback while manipulating tissues, and counter-intuitive movements [4, 5]. In addition, surgeons are often exposed to physical strains from standing in non-comfortable positions for extended periods of time. These difficulties can significantly amplify the complexity of surgical procedures and their outcome.

In more recent years, robotic-assisted surgery has emerged as a new minimal-invasive approach to surgery, integrating current technological advancements in 'traditional' MIS. The concept of robotic-assisted surgery is to enable the surgeon to control the laparoscopic/thoracoscopic instrumentation through a robotic device that is connected to a remote console. Using this technology allows for three-dimensional optics, enhanced range of intuitive instrument motions (even more than the normal open situation), and improved ergonomics [3, 6]. This type of robotic-assisted surgery first gained prominence in the field of urology, mainly for performing radical prostatectomy and complex bladder operations [7]. Since its introduction, the applications for surgical robots has expanded into almost all surgical fields, resulting in its current wide-scale use. For thoracic and vascular surgeons, a growing number of studies have shown that robotic-assisted surgery is feasible and results in favourable outcomes as well [4, 8]. These benefits have mainly been shown in the field of mediastinal tumours and lung cancer surgery, however, the efficacy of robotic-assisted surgery has also been proven for other thoracic and vascular procedures such as first-rib resection, sympathectomy, diaphragmatic paralysis, median arcuate ligament release, and aorto/ilio-femoral bypass surgery for occlusive disease [4, 9].

Despite these advantages and the increasing popularity of these robotic-assisted approaches, there are still controversies regarding the implementation and the use of these approaches, such as the generally high operating costs, lack of haptic feedback, the size of the system, and longer total operative times due to installation of the robotic system [7, 10]. Furthermore, there is a lack of definite data from large prospective studies comparing short-term and long-term outcomes of open surgery with 'traditional' MIS and robotic-assisted surgery in all aspects, including the ergonomics for the surgeon. Nevertheless, these studies are necessary to truly demonstrate the effectiveness and superior outcomes of these emerging surgical approaches. In this chapter review, we summarise the latest data on surgical techniques and treatment outcomes for robotic-assisted thoracic and vascular surgery.

## 2. Robotic-assisted thoracic surgery

In the field of thoracic surgery, video-assisted thoracoscopic surgery (VATS) remains the gold standard approach for thoracic surgery, and it is performed for almost all thoracic surgical indications [4]. In the last few years, robotic-assisted thoracoscopic surgery (RATS) has gained popularity as alternative to VATS due to the flexibility of its endo-wrist instruments, the three-dimensional visualisation, and the more precise and intuitive movements [1, 11]. The majority of studies comparing RATS to VATS and/or thoracotomy have been performed in the field of thoracic oncology, in which the benefits of RATS have already largely been established [12]. However, there is an increasing amount of studies that show similar benefits of RATS in other (non-oncological) thoracic surgical procedures [13]. In this section, we will highlight and review the most commonly performed oncological and non-oncological RATS procedures.

### 2.1 Lung cancer surgery

Lung cancer is worldwide the most common malignancy and one of the leading causes of cancer-related deaths [14]. Despite the widespread implementation of measures mitigating tobacco use, an overall increase in new cases of non-small cell lung cancer (NSCLC) has been noted, mainly due to rising incidence rates in developing countries [15]. The majority of these new lung cancer cases are diagnosed during advanced stages, resulting in low overall five-year survival rates [14]. In these advanced stages, treatment modalities are limited and have minimal effects on overall and disease-free survival. However, due to advancements in diagnostic techniques and imaging modalities, an increasing number of NSCLCs are being detected at earlier stages of disease [16]. In the near future, the number of newly-diagnosed early stage lung cancers will likely increase due to the implementation of lung cancer screening programmes. The NELSON-trial and the NLST-trial have both shown that screening patients with high-risks of developing lung cancer with low-dose chest computed tomography (CT) scans results in significantly lower mortality rates due to earlier cancer detection [17, 18].

For early-stage NSCLC, the gold standard remains surgical management by means of lobectomy with hilar and mediastinal lymph node dissection [19, 20]. Currently, VATS lobectomy is the technique of choice for this procedure as several large-scale studies have shown that VATS results in fewer perioperative complications, less pain, and faster recovery times compared to the traditional open approach [21, 22]. However, in the last decade, RATS has been gaining popularity as a minimal invasive approach due to its ability to overcome the previously described drawbacks of conventional VATS [12]. Despite a lack of well-powered randomised controlled trials comparing RATS to VATS or open surgery for the treatment of (early stage) lung cancer, a growing body of literature has demonstrated a clear advantage of lobectomy by RATS over thoracotomy regarding perioperative blood loss, postoperative analgesia need, postoperative recovery, hospital length of stay (LOS), and 30-day mortality rates [13]. In contrast, results from studies comparing RATS to VATS are less conclusive and, often, contradictory. In a recent meta-analysis of 3239 patients comparing RATS to VATS, a lower 30-day mortality and conversion rate to open surgery was seen in favour of RATS [23]. Similar studies have also shown improved survival rates, fewer postoperative complications, and shorter hospital stays for RATS compared to VATS [24]. However, in a propensity-matched analysis by Oh et al., no difference in mortality was detected between VATS and RATS [25]. Similarly, no significant difference in survival was found in the database analysis of the Society of Thoracic Surgeons (STS) which included 1220 RATS and 12378 VATS lobectomies [26].

Regarding oncological outcomes, only a limited number of studies have been performed comparing RATS to open surgery and/or VATS. There is evidence suggesting that RATS results in increased rates of nodal upstaging and yields higher numbers of nodal stations sampled. However, in a recent data analysis by Hennon et al., 64,676 patients with NSCLC from the National Cancer Database (NCDB) in the USA were analysed for lymph node yield and nodal upstaging. The results of their study did not show any significant difference between the three approaches. The authors concluded that both RATS and VATS are non-inferior to open thoracotomy for intraoperative lymph node evaluation [27]. In addition to the possible benefits regarding treatment and oncological outcomes for lobectomies, an increasing number of experts are advocating for the use of RATS in sublobar resections. For elderly patients, patients with comorbidities, or patients with limited pulmonary reserve, sublobar resections such as wedge resections and segmentectomies have been proposed as viable alternatives [11, 28]. Despite efforts to compare the oncological and survival outcomes of sublobar resections to lobectomy, there is still no clear consensus on whether sublobar resections are indeed non-inferior to lobectomy. Some authors suggest that sublobar resections result in lower overall survival rates, higher positive resection margins, higher recurrence rates, and inadequate lymph node sampling [29]. However, there is a growing number of studies suggesting that segmentectomy has similar overall and disease-free survival rates as lobectomy [30]. Furthermore, sublobar resections have also been associated with improved postoperative quality of life (QoL) [16]. For robotic segmentectomy, the current data suggests that treatment outcomes and complication rates are similar to VATS. In a recent retrospective study by Xie et al., 215 patients that underwent atypical or anatomical segmentectomy by RATS or VATS were analysed for short-term treatment outcomes. The authors concluded that RATS was a safe approach and even resulted in higher lymph node sampling rates and fewer postoperative complications compared to VATS [31].

Even for treating centrally located NSCLC lesions, emerging evidence is suggesting that RATS may play a major role in the near future. A recent retrospective study by Qiu et al. compared treatment and oncological outcomes of RATS to VATS and open surgery in 188 patients undergoing sleeve lobectomy for centrally located NSCLC. RATS was non-inferior to both VATS and open surgery regarding oncological prognosis. However, the robotic group had significantly less blood loss, shorter operative times, and reduced tube drainage times compared to the two other groups. The authors concluded that robotic sleeve lobectomy is a safe, feasible and effective procedure for centrally located NSCLC [32]. Despite all these promising studies, these findings have not been demonstrated in large prospective series or randomised controlled trials (RCT).

### 2.2 Mediastinal masses

Mediastinal masses in the anterior, middle or posterior compartment are a heterogeneous group that account for approximately 3% of all thoracic lesions. The most common mediastinal masses are thymomas, bronchogenic cysts, neurogenic tumours, and thyroid masses. These lesions derive from different germ layers located in various parts of the thoracic cavity [33]. In the past, surgical removal of these mediastinal masses was generally performed using a median sternotomy, posterolateral thoracotomy, or hemi-clamshell sternotomy, often resulting in significant postoperative morbidity [34]. However, the increasingly widespread use of minimal-invasive approaches in other surgical domains has resulted in a similar shift in treatment approaches for mediastinal tumours [35]. Thoracoscopic thymectomy was first described in 1993 and VATS has since become one of the standard approaches for thymic and non-thymic malignancies [35]. Earlier studies have shown that VATS is associated with less perioperative blood loss, shorter operation times, and less chest tube drainage compared to open procedures [36]. In the past two decades, robotic surgery has gained popularity in the treatment of mediastinal masses as well. Similar to the situation for lung cancer surgery, RATS has advantages over conventional VATS due to its three-dimensional image and multi-articulated instruments, providing easy access to the small mediastinal space and allowing safe removal of mediastinal masses [37, 38]. While comparisons of treatment outcomes and postoperative complications between open and MIS approaches have been performed before, few studies have directly compared VATS to RATS for mediastinal masses.

In a retrospective study by Qian et al., 123 patients with early-stage thymoma were analysed to compare treatment outcomes for VATS, RATS, and median sternotomy. The authors concluded that RATS and VATS are both feasible techniques for early-stage thymomas with similar oncological outcomes compared to open surgery. However, their data did show more favourable outcomes for RATS regarding post-operative pleural drainage duration time, drainage volumes, and hospital LOS [39]. Other recent studies have corroborated these findings as well. Zeng et al. retrospectively analysed 274 patients that underwent multiportal VATS, uniportal VATS, or RATS resection of a mediastinal mass. Compared with multiportal VATS, uniportal VATS and RATS had a significantly shorter chest tube placement time and hospital LOS without increasing the incidence rate of complications. The RATS approach was associated with better intraoperative safety and was considered non-inferior regarding postoperative outcomes compared to multiportal VATS [40]. In a very recent retrospective cohort study using the National Inpatient Sample (NIS) database, an estimated total of 23,087 patients that underwent thymectomy were included to compare outcomes after open, VATS, and RATS thymectomy. The majority of patients were treated for thymoma or myasthenia gravis, with approximately 16,025 patients (69%) in the open surgery group, 4,119 (18%) in the VATS group, and 3,097 (13%) in the RATS group. In the analysed period of 2008–2014, trend analysis revealed a decline in open surgery, while the performance of VATS and RATS had increased. No significant differences in overall complication rates or hospital LOS were found in this study. However, RATS was associated with lower rates of cardiac complications and haemorrhage [41]. Even for the rarer posterior mediastinal tumours, recent data suggests that RATS may be superior in terms of postoperative blood loss and hospital LOS compared to VATS [4].

### 2.3 First rib resection

Thoracic outlet syndrome (TOS) is a complex disorder that comprises a myriad of possible symptoms which arise from compression of the brachial plexus, subclavian artery, and/or the subclavian vein. This compression generally occurs in the triangular space referred to as the thoracic outlet, which is located between the first rib, the clavicle, and the scalene muscles [42]. The majority of patients with TOS can be treated with non-surgical measures such as medication, posture correction, physical therapy, or taping. However, in a relatively small number of patients, these conservative treatments fail to alleviate the symptoms, often resulting in significant morbidity [43]. In these patients, or when vascular structures are involved, surgical decompression with removal of the first rib is usually necessary. Over the last decades, several types of surgical approaches and techniques have been described. Historically, extrathoracic approaches have used a supraclavicular or transaxillary incision to resect the first rib. Despite their well-documented effectiveness, many authors have asserted that these approaches are regularly associated with complications such as brachial plexus injury or vascular injury [44].

The intrathoracic approach using VATS has been the most popular approach in the last decade, owing to the theoretical advantage of fewer postoperative neurovascular complications and incomplete resections [45]. In recent years, the robotic-assisted approach has rapidly gained ground as a viable alternative to VATS due to its superior optics and instrument control [44]. However, this remains a relatively new field with only a limited number of studies published reporting outcomes of RATS first rib resections. Data from retrospective studies and case series from the last decade suggests that the robotic approach is safe, effective, and non-inferior to the VATS approach [46]. In a recent single-center, prospective study by Burt et al. RATS first rib resection was compared to the conventional supraclavicular approach in 116 patients (66 RATS and 50 open surgery). Postoperative pain and analgesia need was significantly lower in the robotic approach group. Furthermore, RATS was associated with fewer cases of brachial plexus palsy and overall complication rates [47]. Despite these promising results, there is still a lack of data from larger, prospective studies comparing RATS, VATS, and open approaches for first rib resections.

### 2.4 Sympathectomy

Presently, hyperhidrosis is the main indication for sympathectomy, which can be performed through various surgical approaches, such as the posterior thoracic approach, transaxillary approach, transthoracic approach, VATS approach, and RATS approach. The sympathectomy itself is usually performed by ganglionectomy, clipping, or ablation of the dorsal sympathetic chain [48]. The extent to which the sympathectomy is performed is a controversial subject as it is correlated to the incidence of complications. More extended sympathectomy has been associated with higher rates of compensatory hyperhidrosis. Despite a lack of clear guidelines, the general consensus is to perform an interruption of T3 and T4 for palmar hyperhidrosis, and interruption of T4 and T5 palmar and axillary or palmar, axillary, and pedal hyperhidrosis [49].

A more precise variation of this technique is the selective postganglionic sympathectomy, which involves an interruption of only the postganglionic rami, leaving the sympathetic trunk and ganglia intact. The branches accompanying intercostal nerves 2–4 to the upper extremities are interrupted selectively [50]. Previous studies have shown that this technique of selective postganglionic sympathectomy has success rates up to 95% with only minimal rates of compensatory hyperhidrosis [51]. Only limited data is available regarding robotic selective sympathectomy. However, data from single-institution case series have shown that robotic-assisted selective (postganglionic) sympathectomy is a safe technique with favourable results [52, 53]. In a recent prospective case series by Gharagozloo et al., a total of 47 patients underwent two-staged bilateral robotic selective dorsal preganglionic and postganglionic sympathectomy. Their data showed excellent relief of hyperhidrosis, and minimal rates of compensatory hyperhidrosis and complications. The authors used a two-staged approach to allow the transient compensatory hyperhidrosis to dissipate and to obviate postoperative thoracic pain due to the use of robotic ports [48]. Despite a lack of larger prospective and randomised trials, the current evidence suggests that the robotic-assisted approach has the potential of accomplishing hyperselective sympathectomy with accuracy and minimal rates of compensatory hyperhidrosis and complications such as Horner's syndrome.

### 2.5 Diaphragmatic plication

Diaphragmatic paralysis is an uncommon condition that is characterised by elevation of a hemidiaphragm. If symptomatic, patients often experience dyspnoea during exercise, orthopnoea, fatigue, insomnia, and an overall reduced quality of life. In adult patients, the most common causes of diaphragmatic paralysis are idiopathic, tumour invasion of the phrenic nerve, or damage to the phrenic nerve during cardiothoracic surgery [54]. Surgical treatment is indicated exclusively for symptomatic patients, and the preferred surgical technique is (hemi)diaphragmatic plication [55]. The traditional method is the open transthoracic plication, and is still widely used today. However, an increasing number of surgeons are moving towards less invasive approaches such as laparoscopy or thoracoscopy. VATS diaphragm plication has already demonstrated to be a safe and feasible technique for symptomatic patients [56, 57]. However, technical difficulties due to the limited workspace in the thorax and the elevated hemidiaphragm often lead to the adoption of a (mini)thoracotomy. Robotic-assisted surgery offers all the benefits of MIS while simultaneously providing the surgeon the same dexterity as the open approach. Several case studies and small case-series have reported excellent outcomes with the robotic approach for diaphragmatic plication [58, 59]. However, robust and conclusive data regarding long-term outcomes are still missing.

## 3. Robotic-assisted vascular surgery

In the last few decades, the field of vascular surgery has changed dramatically with the introduction of endovascular surgery. There has been a significant paradigm shift towards these endovascular approaches for the treatment of a wide array of venous and arterial diseases [8]. However, despite the fact that many vascular surgeons have been willing to embrace innovative, minimally-invasive techniques, the implementation of laparoscopic vascular surgery has only been a relatively minor success. This has mainly been due to the difficulties associated with laparoscopic vascular surgery such as the suturing of vascular anastomoses and long clamping times [9]. Furthermore, for an increasingly large number of procedures, an endovascular technique has been developed. However, with the advent of robotic-assisted approaches, new opportunities have risen for vascular surgeons, especially for disease states that are not amenable to endovascular interventions and for which current approaches are technically challenging or associated with significant morbidity. In this section, we will discuss the latest data regarding indications and outcomes of robotic-assisted vascular surgery.

### 3.1 Median arcuate ligament release

Median arcuate ligament syndrome (MALS) is caused by compression of the celiac artery and plexus by the median arcuate ligament of the diaphragmatic crura [60]. In a normal population, the median arcuate ligament crosses the aorta anteriorly above the celiac origin between levels T11 and L1. However, in approximately 12–49% of the population, an anatomic variant exists in which the ligament passes inferiorly, causing compression of the celiac artery and ganglion. The majority of patients with this anatomical variant are asymptomatic due to a rich network of collateral vessels between the celiac and superior mesenteric arteries. However, a number of patients do develop symptoms despite the presence of collateral arteries, frequently presenting with a variety of abdominal symptoms including nausea, vomiting, postprandial epigastric pain, and weight loss [61]. Over the years, several different interventions have been proposed for symptomatic MALS using different approaches such as open surgery, laparoscopic surgery, endovascular angioplasty, or hybrid procedures combining laparoscopic and endovascular techniques [60]. Surgical release of the extrinsic compression caused by the median arcuate ligament remains the mainstay of therapy, with overall success rates ranging from 53 to 79% and a majority of patients reporting rapid postoperative symptom relief [62].

In more recent years, the robotic approach has been gaining popularity due to its technical advantages over conventional laparoscopic surgery. In 2007, Jaik et al. were the first to report a robotic-assisted MALR [63]. Since then, several other case series have been published. In a case series of 13 patients, Khrucharoen et al. analysed outcomes symptomatic patients undergoing robotic-assisted MALR. The authors found that robotic-assisted MALR is safe and feasible in selected patients an may be associated with reduced operative times [61]. In a follow-up study by the same group, laparoscopic and robotic-assisted MALR were compared for short- and intermediate-term clinical outcomes. In their retrospective study, a total of 34 patients were included (16 laparoscopic and 18 robotic cases) for further analysis.

Complete pain resolution was achieved in 37.5% in the laparoscopic group and in 44.4% in the robotic group ($p = 0.93$). The data showed no difference between conversion rates to open surgery, symptom recurrence rates, postoperative pain, and overall clinical improvement. However, median operative time was significantly shorter in the robotic group compared to the open group (179.5 versus 106 minutes, $p < 0.001$). The authors concluded that both laparoscopic and robotic-assisted MALR offer similar short- and intermediate-term outcomes, with a possible shorter operative time achievable by a robotic-assisted approach [64]. In another recent retrospective study by Fernstrum et al., 27 patients that underwent robotic MALR were included for analysis. Long-term improvement or resolution of symptoms and symptom recurrence was used as primary outcome. Their data showed mean operative times of 95 minutes and two cases of conversion to open surgery. Only one major complication occurred, which was an inadvertent arteriotomy of the celiac trunk that occurred while dividing a portion of the diaphragmatic fibres. After more than 30 days follow-up, 68% of patients had full symptom relief and 4% had partial symptom resolution. Furthermore, 4% of patients had no symptom resolution and 24% had symptom recurrence after an initial period of symptom resolution. The authors concluded that robotic MALR is a safe option for treatment of MALS with high-response rates [65].

### 3.2 Vascular bypass surgery

Aortoiliac occlusive disease (AIOD) can result in symptoms such as claudication and critical ischemia of the lower extremities. Generally, AIOD is treated by either endovascular or open surgery, depending on the severity and location of the occlusion. Whereas for extensive AIOD patients are generally treated using an open approach, endovascular approaches with covered stents have also been introduced with success using the 'covered endovascular reconstruction of aortic bifurcation (CERAB) technique [66]. The main disadvantage of endovascular repair are the high costs for the patient, insurance companies or hospitals [67]. An alternative for open surgery or endovascular therapy is a laparoscopic reconstruction [68]. A number of laparoscopic techniques for treating AIOD have been developed over the last few years with the aim of reducing operative trauma and achieving faster postoperative recovery rates. However, performing laparoscopic aortic surgery and vascular anastomoses is very challenging and requires intensive training [69]. More recently, robotic-assisted approaches have been developed in order to overcome these limitations of the conventional laparoscopic approach. In a retrospective case-series by Jongkind et al., a total of 28 patients that underwent robotic-assisted laparoscopic surgery (RALS) for AIOD were included. In this group, 24 patients received robotic-assisted laparoscopic aortobifemoral bypass grafting and 4 patients received an aortoiliac endarterectomy. Their results showed a median operative time of 350 minutes and median aortic clamping time of 70 minutes. In 4 patients, conversion to open surgery was necessary. One patient died within 30 days postoperatively and 4 patients had non-lethal complications. The authors concluded that RALS is a feasible and durable technique for treating patients with AIOD [70].

Other studies and case series have found similar clinical outcomes and complication rates. In another relatively recent retrospective study, 310 patients that underwent robotic-assisted vascular surgery were included for analysis. In this patient population, 224 patients underwent robotic-assisted surgery for treatment of occlusive disease, which included robotic ilio-femoral bypass, aorto-femoral bypass, and aorto-iliac thromboendarterectomy with prosthetic patch. Median clamping time and anastomosis times were 37 and 24 minutes, respectively. Mean total operative time was 194 minutes. In 2 cases (0.9%), a conversion to open surgery was necessary. Lastly, median hospital LOS was 5 days. The authors concluded that the greatest advantage of these robotic-assisted procedures was the speed and relative ease with which vascular anastomoses could be performed [9]. This offers significant benefits regarding temporary lower limb ischemia times during aortic clamping. Despite the lack of large-scale clinical studies, the currently available data suggests that robotic-assisted approaches can play a significant role in treating arterial occlusive disease. These robotic approaches can even be combined with endovascular or open approaches into hybrid procedures, thus making it a versatile and potentially useful tool for the modern vascular surgeon.

### 3.3 Aortic aneurysm surgery

One of the greatest paradigm shifts towards MIS in the last decade has taken place in the field to the of aortic aneurysm surgery. With the introduction of endovascular approaches, the number of open aneurysm repairs has decreased dramatically, having steadily been replaced by endovascular aneurysm repair (EVAR) [71, 72]. Nevertheless, for patients that do not qualify for endovascular repair or with complications following endovascular repair, surgical repair of the aneurysm is often necessary. For this subset of patients, a minimal invasive approach may be an appealing alternative to the conventional open repair. Although laparoscopic techniques have been described for aortic aneurysm repair, this approach remains somewhat unappealing to many surgeons due to the steep learning curve [71]. Another possibility is the robotic-assisted approach for aneurysm repair, which is able to overcome the kinematics limitations of laparoscopy. Previous retrospective studies and case series have already shown the feasibility of the robotic approach for several types of aortic aneurysm repairs.

In a study by Stádler et al., 65 patients that underwent robotic-assisted aorto-iliac aneurysm surgery were included in a retrospective analysis of outcomes after robotic-assisted vascular procedures. Median operative time and aortic cross clamping time were 253 and 93 minutes, respectively. Overall mortality was 1.6%, median conversion rate was 13%, and no major non-lethal postoperative complications were noted. Furthermore, median hospital LOS was 7 days. The results regarding operative times and outcomes are similar to the conventional open repair technique, with the added benefits of MIS [9]. In addition to this, robotic-assisted surgery could also have a specific role in type-II endoleaks, the most frequent complication after EVAR. Currently these types of leaks are treated with surgical ligation or endovascular embolization, the latter being the first-line treatment option. However, endovascular embolizations of endoleaks has high recurrence rates. With the robotic approach, these endoleaks can be repaired more easily than with a laparoscopic approach, while simultaneously providing a more definitive solution for the endoleak. Morelli et al. showed that this technique is feasible in their recent case series [73].

## 4. Costs of robotic surgery

Despite the increasing popularity of robotic-assisted approaches worldwide, concerns have been raised regarding the high costs of acquiring and maintaining robotic systems [16]. In addition, stapling devices in robotic surgery often come at a high price, necessitating many centres to use standard manual or electronic stapling devices by the table surgeon instead of the console surgeon. Several studies have attempted to perform cost-analysis studies of robotic surgery compared to open and laparoscopic/thoracoscopic approaches. However, there are often significant discrepancies between these studies, mainly due to different definitions of cost (console and robot; maintenance; instruments; stapling devices) and differences in healthcare and insurance regulations between countries [10]. A large-scale analysis of the NIS database showed that median costs of RATS were significantly higher than conventional VATS [74]. Similar findings were reported in an analysis of the Premier registry by Swanson et al. However, there is evidence to suggest that RATS is comparable or even less expensive than open surgery, mainly due to reduced operative times and shorter hospital LOS [75]. Furthermore, previous studies have shown that as programmes adopt and perform more robotic operations, the overall costs of hospitalisation will decrease [71]. These costs will likely decrease even more over time with the introduction of upcoming competitors' surgical robotic platforms [1].

## 5. Ergonomics of robotic surgery

In addition to the patient-related benefits of robotic surgery, these robotic platforms allow for a more ergonomic working environment for the surgeon [16]. Previous studies have already shown that work-related musculoskeletal disorders are frequently encountered among surgeons and surgical residents [76]. This is a result of several factors, such as frequent repetitive movements of the trunk and upper extremities and prolonged static body positioning [77]. When these work-related musculoskeletal disorders are not corrected early on, they can result in injuries such as carpal tunnel syndrome, wrist tendonitis, chronic back and knee pain, TOS, and the development of varicose veins [76, 78]. Several studies have compared conventional laparoscopic and robotic approaches and have found that surgeons using robotic surgery report less overall pain [79, 80]. In addition, data has shown that ergonomic training courses for surgeons can also significantly reduce pain [77]. However, more robust data from larger studies are necessary to measure the effect of robotic surgery on ergonomics, and physical and mental fatigue compared to conventional approaches.

## 6. Future of robotic surgery

Since the introduction of robotic-assisted surgery, surgeons and medical engineers have continuously searched for new technologies and advancements across all surgical fields. Since its introduction approximately 20 years ago, the da Vinci robotic surgery system (Intuitive Surgical Inc., Sunnyvale, CA, USA) has been involved in over 5 million operations, making Intuitive Surgical the largest player in the surgical robotic market [81]. However, with the original da Vinci patents now expiring, many medical 'tech' companies are now setting their sights on joining this lucrative, growing market. New systems in the near future will likely aim to improve on the current robotic models by incorporating new technologies such as single-port instrumental arms, haptic feedback, eye-movement tracking, and virtual reality (VR) [82]. In addition to the technological aspects of the current robotic systems, there are also some important practical limitations that can be improved upon, such as the high operational costs, the size of the robotic systems, and its accessibility in lower-income countries. Several "large" robotic systems have become available in the last few years. Some examples are the Senhance console (TransEnterix, Morrisville, NC, USA), BITRACK system (Rob Surgical, Barcelona, Spain), and the Revo-i surgical robot (Meere Company, Seoul, South Korea). These systems each have some advantages over the da Vinci system, such as haptic feedback or eye-tracking, but are generally limited by their price and large size [81].

In addition to these large systems, many companies have started to create smaller, more portable systems that allow more flexibility in hospitals that do not have robot-dedicated operating rooms. Perhaps the most daring and revolutionary concept that is entering the field of surgery is the surgical microrobot. Microrobot surgery is fundamentally different to the current robotic systems as it is not physically tethered to a console. These microbots can be propelled externally via electromagnetic fields or ultrasonographic energy, or internally using chemical reactions. Recent proof-of-concepts have shown that these microbots are able to perform various surgical manoeuvres such as dissecting, grasping, and ablation at a microscale [83–85]. Undoubtedly, the future of robotic surgery looks exciting as many new technologies are emerging at an exponential pace. The COVID-19 pandemic has shown an unprecedented demand of surgical robotic systems as well, mainly due to their ability of providing an additional shielding layer between the healthcare worker and the patient [86]. It is likely that this demand will outlast the pandemic itself and propel the development of surgical robotic technology.

## 7. Conclusion

It is without a doubt that robotic surgery has changed the surgical world over the last decade. An increasingly large group of surgeons are incorporating robotic approaches in their daily practice as more and more data has shown the benefits of these approaches. In thoracic surgery, RATS has proven to be a valuable tool for many oncological and non-oncological indications, resulting in it being considered one of the standard treatment approaches in many centres. Similar, although less prominent, trends are being noted in the field of vascular surgery as well. However, despite these promising future perspectives, there is still a lack of well-powered, multi-centre randomised trials comparing robotic approaches to open surgery or conventional laparoscopy/thoracoscopy. Furthermore, more data regarding the cost and cost efficiency of robotic surgery are necessary in order to determine whether the benefits of robotic-assisted approaches outweigh its costs.

## Conflict of interest

The authors declare no conflict of interest.

## Author details

Lawek Berzenji, Krishan Yogeswaran, Patrick Lauwers, Paul Van Schil and Jeroen M.H. Hendriks*
Department of Thoracic and Vascular Surgery, Antwerp University Hospital, Antwerp, Belgium

*Address all correspondence to: jeroen.hendriks@uza.be

## References

[1] Diana M, Marescaux J. Robotic surgery. Br J Surg 2015;102;e15–e28.

[2] Power AD, D'Souza DM, Moffatt-Bruce SD, Merritt RE, Kneuertz PJ. Defining the learning curve of robotic thoracic surgery: what does it take? Surg Endosc 2019;33;3880-3888.

[3] Wright JD. Robotic-Assisted Surgery: Balancing Evidence and Implementation. JAMA 2017;318;1545-1547.

[4] Cosgun T, Kaba E, Ayalp K, Alomari MR, Toker A. Robot-Assisted Thoracoscopic Surgery: Pros and Cons. Current Surgery Reports 2017;5;27.

[5] Abbas AE. Surgical Management of Lung Cancer: History, Evolution, and Modern Advances. Curr Oncol Rep 2018;20;98.

[6] Rajaram R, Mohanty S, Bentrem DJ, Pavey ES, Odell DD, Bharat A, et al. Nationwide Assessment of Robotic Lobectomy for Non-Small Cell Lung Cancer. Ann Thorac Surg 2017;103;1092-1100.

[7] Hu JC, Gu X, Lipsitz SR, Barry MJ, D'Amico AV, Weinberg AC, et al. Comparative effectiveness of minimally invasive vs open radical prostatectomy. JAMA 2009;302;1557-1564.

[8] Miller K, Bergman D, Stante G, Vemuri C. Exploration of robotic-assisted surgical techniques in vascular surgery. J Robot Surg 2019;13;689-693.

[9] Stadler P, Dvoracek L, Vitasek P, Matous P. Robot assisted Aortic and Non-aortic Vascular Operations. Eur J Vasc Endovasc Surg 2016;52;22-28.

[10] Singer E, Kneuertz PJ, D'Souza DM, Moffatt-Bruce SD, Merritt RE. Understanding the financial cost of robotic lobectomy: calculating the value of innovation? Ann Cardiothorac Surg 2019;8;194-201.

[11] Veronesi G. Robotic lobectomy and segmentectomy for lung cancer: results and operating technique. J Thorac Dis 2015;7;S122–S130.

[12] Velez-Cubian FO, Ng EP, Fontaine JP, Toloza EM. Robotic-Assisted Videothoracoscopic Surgery of the Lung. Cancer Control 2015;22;314-325.

[13] Zirafa CC, Romano G, Key TH, Davini F, Melfi F. The evolution of robotic thoracic surgery. Annals of Cardiothoracic Surgery 2019;8;210-217.

[14] Wong MCS, Lao XQ, Ho KF, Goggins WB, Tse SLA. Incidence and mortality of lung cancer: global trends and association with socioeconomic status. Sci Rep 2017;7;14300.

[15] Malvezzi M, Carioli G, Bertuccio P, Boffetta P, Levi F, La Vecchia C, et al. European cancer mortality predictions for the year 2017, with focus on lung cancer. Ann Oncol 2017;28;1117-1123.

[16] Berzenji L, Yogeswaran K, Van Schil P, Lauwers P, Hendriks JMH. Use of Robotics in Surgical Treatment of Non-small Cell Lung Cancer. Curr Treat Options Oncol 2020;21;80.

[17] de Koning HJ, van der Aalst CM, de Jong PA, Scholten ET, Nackaerts K, Heuvelmans MA, et al. Reduced Lung-Cancer Mortality with Volume CT Screening in a Randomized Trial. New England Journal of Medicine 2020;382;503-513.

[18] Lung Cancer Incidence and Mortality with Extended Follow-up in the National Lung Screening Trial. Journal of Thoracic Oncology 2019;14;1732-1742.

[19] Ginsberg RJ, Rubinstein LV. Randomized trial of lobectomy versus limited resection for T1 N0 non-small cell lung cancer. Lung Cancer Study Group. Ann Thorac Surg 1995;60; 615-622; discussion 22-3.

[20] Lang-Lazdunski L. Surgery for nonsmall cell lung cancer. Eur Respir Rev 2013;22;382-404.

[21] Ujiie H, Gregor A, Yasufuku K. Minimally invasive surgical approaches for lung cancer. Expert Rev Respir Med 2019;13;571-578.

[22] Ikeda N. Updates on Minimally Invasive Surgery in Non-Small Cell Lung Cancer. Curr Treat Options Oncol 2019;20;16.

[23] Liang H, Liang W, Zhao L, Chen D, Zhang J, Zhang Y, et al. Robotic Versus Video-assisted Lobectomy/ Segmentectomy for Lung Cancer: A Meta-analysis. Ann Surg 2018;268;254-259.

[24] Emmert A, Straube C, Buentzel J, Roever C. Robotic versus thoracoscopic lung resection: A systematic review and meta-analysis. Medicine (Baltimore) 2017;96;e7633.

[25] Oh DS, Reddy RM, Gorrepati ML, Mehendale S, Reed MF. Robotic-Assisted, Video-Assisted Thoracoscopic and Open Lobectomy: Propensity-Matched Analysis of Recent Premier Data. Ann Thorac Surg 2017;104;1733-1740.

[26] Louie BE, Wilson JL, Kim S, Cerfolio RJ, Park BJ, Farivar AS, et al. Comparison of Video-Assisted Thoracoscopic Surgery and Robotic Approaches for Clinical Stage I and Stage II Non-Small Cell Lung Cancer Using The Society of Thoracic Surgeons Database. Ann Thorac Surg 2016;102;917-924.

[27] Hennon MW, DeGraaff LH, Groman A, Demmy TL, Yendamuri S. The association of nodal upstaging with surgical approach and its impact on long-term survival after resection of non-small-cell lung cancer. Eur J Cardiothorac Surg 2020;57;888-895.

[28] Detterbeck FC. Lobectomy versus limited resection in T1N0 lung cancer. Ann Thorac Surg 2013;96;742-744.

[29] Khullar OV, Liu Y, Gillespie T, Higgins KA, Ramalingam S, Lipscomb J, et al. Survival After Sublobar Resection versus Lobectomy for Clinical Stage IA Lung Cancer: An Analysis from the National Cancer Data Base. J Thorac Oncol 2015;10;1625-1633.

[30] Cao C, Gupta S, Chandrakumar D, Tian DH, Black D, Yan TD. Meta-analysis of intentional sublobar resections versus lobectomy for early stage non-small cell lung cancer. Ann Cardiothorac Surg 2014;3;134-141.

[31] Xie B, Sun X, Qin Y, Liu A, Miao S, Jiao W. Short-term outcomes of typical versus atypical lung segmentectomy by minimally invasive surgeries. Thorac Cancer 2019;10;1812-1818.

[32] Qiu T, Zhao Y, Xuan Y, Qin Y, Niu Z, Shen Y, et al. Robotic sleeve lobectomy for centrally located non-small cell lung cancer: A propensity score-weighted comparison with thoracoscopic and open surgery. J Thorac Cardiovasc Surg 2020;160;838-46.e2.

[33] Chen K, Zhang X, Jin R, Xiang J, Han D, Zhang Y, et al. Robot-assisted thoracoscopic surgery for mediastinal masses: a single-institution experience. J Thorac Dis 2020;12;105-113.

[34] Davenport E, Malthaner RA. The role of surgery in the management of thymoma: a systematic review. Ann Thorac Surg 2008;86;673-684.

[35] Ropper AH. RetroSternal--Looking Back at Thymectomy for Myasthenia Gravis. N Engl J Med 2016;375;576-577.

[36] Hess NR, Sarkaria IS, Pennathur A, Levy RM, Christie NA, Luketich JD. Minimally invasive versus open thymectomy: a systematic review of surgical techniques, patient demographics, and perioperative outcomes. Ann Cardiothorac Surg 2016;5;1-9.

[37] Curcio C, Scaramuzzi R, Amore D. Robotic-assisted thoracoscopic surgery thymectomy. J Vis Surg 2017;3;162.

[38] Li F, Ismail M, Elsner A, Uluk D, Bauer G, Meisel A, et al. Surgical Techniques for Myasthenia Gravis: Robotic-Assisted Thoracoscopic Surgery. Thorac Surg Clin 2019;29;177-186.

[39] Qian L, Chen X, Huang J, Lin H, Mao F, Zhao X, et al. A comparison of three approaches for the treatment of early-stage thymomas: robot-assisted thoracic surgery, video-assisted thoracic surgery, and median sternotomy. J Thorac Dis 2017;9;1997-2005.

[40] Zeng L, Wang W, Han J, Zhu L, Zhao J, Tu Z. Uniportal video-assisted thoracoscopic surgery and robot-assisted thoracoscopic surgery are feasible approaches with potential advantages in minimally invasive mediastinal lesions resection. Gland surgery 2021;10;101-111.

[41] Seo YJ, Christian-Miller N, Aguayo E, Sanaiha Y, Benharash P, Yanagawa J. National Utilization and Short-Term Outcomes of Video and Robot-assisted Thoracoscopic Thymectomies. Ann Thorac Surg 2021.

[42] Peek J, Vos CG, Unlu C, van de Pavoordt H, van den Akker PJ, de Vries JPM. Outcome of Surgical Treatment for Thoracic Outlet Syndrome: Systematic Review and Meta-Analysis. Ann Vasc Surg 2017;40;303-326.

[43] Dua A, Deslarzes-Dubuis C, Rothenberg KA, Gologorsky R, Lee JT. Long-term Functional Outcomes Follow-up after 188 Rib Resections in Patients with TOS. Ann Vasc Surg 2020;68;28-33.

[44] Kocher GJ, Zehnder A, Lutz JA, Schmidli J, Schmid RA. First Rib Resection for Thoracic Outlet Syndrome: The Robotic Approach. World J Surg 2018;42;3250-3255.

[45] Hwang J, Min B-J, Jo W-M, Shin JS. Video-assisted thoracoscopic surgery for intrathoracic first rib resection in thoracic outlet syndrome. Journal of thoracic disease 2017;9;2022-2028.

[46] Jones MR, Prabhakar A, Viswanath O, Urits I, Green JB, Kendrick JB, et al. Thoracic Outlet Syndrome: A Comprehensive Review of Pathophysiology, Diagnosis, and Treatment. Pain Ther 2019;8;5-18.

[47] Burt BM, Palivela N, Cekmecelioglu D, Paily P, Najafi B, Lee H-S, et al. Safety of robotic first rib resection for thoracic outlet syndrome. The Journal of Thoracic and Cardiovascular Surgery.

[48] Gharagozloo F, Meyer M, Tempesta B. Robotic Staged Bilateral Selective Postganglionic Sympathectomy for Upper-Extremity Hyperhidrosis. Surg Technol Int 2020;36;265-269.

[49] Cerfolio RJ, De Campos JR, Bryant AS, Connery CP, Miller DL, DeCamp MM, et al. The Society of Thoracic Surgeons expert consensus for the surgical treatment of hyperhidrosis. Ann Thorac Surg 2011;91;1642-1648.

[50] Lee DY, Kim DH, Paik HC. Selective division of T3 rami communicantes (T3 ramicotomy) in the treatment of palmar hyperhidrosis. Ann Thorac Surg 2004;78;1052-1055.

[51] Friedel G, Linder A, Toomes H. Selective video-assisted thoracoscopic

sympathectomy. Thorac Cardiovasc Surg 1993;41;245-248.

[52] Coveliers H, Meyer M, Gharagozloo F, Wisselink W, Rauwerda J, Margolis M, et al. Robotic selective postganglionic thoracic sympathectomy for the treatment of hyperhidrosis. Ann Thorac Surg 2013;95;269-274.

[53] Coveliers H, Meyer M, Gharagozloo F, Wisselink W. Selective sympathectomy for hyperhidrosis: technique of robotic transthoracic selective postganglionic efferent sympathectomy. Eur J Cardiothorac Surg 2013;43;428-430.

[54] Groth SS, Andrade RS. Diaphragm plication for eventration or paralysis: a review of the literature. Ann Thorac Surg 2010;89;S2146–S2150.

[55] Biswas Roy S, Haworth C, Ipsen T, Kang P, Hill D, Do A, et al. Transabdominal robot-assisted diaphragmatic plication: a 3.5-year experience. European Journal of Cardio-Thoracic Surgery 2017;53;247-253.

[56] Kocher GJ, Zehnder A, Schmid RA. Completely Thoracoscopic Diaphragmatic Plication. World Journal of Surgery 2017;41;1019-1022.

[57] Celik S, Celik M, Aydemir B, Tunckaya C, Okay T, Dogusoy I. Long-term results of diaphragmatic plication in adults with unilateral diaphragm paralysis. Journal of Cardiothoracic Surgery 2010;5;111.

[58] Kwak T, Lazzaro R, Pournik H, Ciaburri D, Tortolani A, Gulkarov I. Robotic thoracoscopic plication for symptomatic diaphragm paralysis. J Robot Surg 2012;6;345-348.

[59] Zwischenberger BA, Kister N, Zwischenberger JB, Martin JT. Laparoscopic Robot-Assisted Diaphragm Plication. The Annals of Thoracic Surgery 2016;101;369-371.

[60] Kim EN, Lamb K, Relles D, Moudgill N, DiMuzio PJ, Eisenberg JA. Median Arcuate Ligament Syndrome-Review of This Rare Disease. JAMA Surg 2016;151;471-477.

[61] Khrucharoen U, Juo YY, Sanaiha Y, Chen Y, Jimenez JC, Dutson EP. Robotic-assisted laparoscopic median arcuate ligament release: 7-year experience from a single tertiary care center. Surg Endosc 2018;32;4029-4035.

[62] Jimenez JC, Harlander-Locke M, Dutson EP. Open and laparoscopic treatment of median arcuate ligament syndrome. J Vasc Surg 2012;56;869-873.

[63] Jaik NP, Stawicki SP, Weger NS, Lukaszczyk JJ. Celiac artery compression syndrome: successful utilization of robotic-assisted laparoscopic approach. J Gastrointestin Liver Dis 2007;16;93-96.

[64] Khrucharoen U, Juo YY, Chen Y, Jimenez JC, Dutson EP. Short- and intermediate-term clinical outcome comparison between laparoscopic and robotic-assisted median arcuate ligament release. J Robot Surg 2020;14;123-129.

[65] Fernstrum C, Pryor M, Wright GP, Wolf AM. Robotic Surgery for Median Arcuate Ligament Syndrome. JSLS 2020;24.

[66] Reijnen MM. Update on covered endovascular reconstruction of the aortic bifurcation. Vascular 2020;28;225-232.

[67] Taeymans K, Goverde P, Lauwers K, Verbruggen P. The CERAB technique: tips, tricks and results. J Cardiovasc Surg (Torino) 2016;57;343-349.

[68] Brown KN, Muco E, Gonzalez L. Leriche Syndrome. StatPearls. Treasure

Island (FL): StatPearls Publishing Copyright © 2021, StatPearls Publishing LLC.; 2021.

[69] Antoniou GA, Riga CV, Mayer EK, Cheshire NJW, Bicknell CD. Clinical applications of robotic technology in vascular and endovascular surgery. Journal of Vascular Surgery 2011;53;493-499.

[70] Jongkind V, Diks J, Yeung KK, Cuesta MA, Wisselink W. Mid-term results of robot-assisted laparoscopic surgery for aortoiliac occlusive disease. Vascular 2011;19;1-7.

[71] Guadagni S, Bianchini M, Palmeri M, Moglia A, Berchiolli RN, Morelli L. HALS, EVAR and robot-assisted surgery as minimally invasive approaches for abdominal aneurysm treatment. J Robot Surg 2020;14;237-238.

[72] Suckow BD, Goodney PP, Columbo JA, Kang R, Stone DH, Sedrakyan A, et al. National trends in open surgical, endovascular, and branched-fenestrated endovascular aortic aneurysm repair in Medicare patients. J Vasc Surg 2018;67;1690-1697 e1.

[73] Morelli L, Guadagni S, Di Franco G, Palmeri M, Furbetta N, Gianardi D, et al. Technical details and preliminary results of a full robotic type II endoleak treatment with the da Vinci Xi. J Robot Surg 2019;13;505-509.

[74] Paul S, Jalbert J, Isaacs AJ, Altorki NK, Isom OW, Sedrakyan A. Comparative effectiveness of robotic-assisted vs thoracoscopic lobectomy. Chest 2014;146;1505-1512.

[75] Swanson SJ, Miller DL, McKenna RJ, Jr., Howington J, Marshall MB, Yoo AC, et al. Comparing robot-assisted thoracic surgical lobectomy with conventional video-assisted thoracic surgical lobectomy and wedge resection: results from a multihospital database (Premier). J Thorac Cardiovasc Surg 2014;147;929-937.

[76] Epstein S, Sparer EH, Tran BN, Ruan QZ, Dennerlein JT, Singhal D, et al. Prevalence of Work-Related Musculoskeletal Disorders Among Surgeons and Interventionalists: A Systematic Review and Meta-analysis. JAMA Surg 2018;153;e174947.

[77] Catanzarite T, Tan-Kim J, Whitcomb EL, Menefee S. Ergonomics in Surgery: A Review. Female Pelvic Med Reconstr Surg 2018;24;1-12.

[78] Yang L, Wang T, Weidner TK, Madura JA, 2nd, Morrow MM, Hallbeck MS. Intraoperative musculoskeletal discomfort and risk for surgeons during open and laparoscopic surgery. Surg Endosc 2020.

[79] van der Schatte Olivier RH, Van't Hullenaar CD, Ruurda JP, Broeders IA. Ergonomics, user comfort, and performance in standard and robot-assisted laparoscopic surgery. Surg Endosc 2009;23;1365-1371.

[80] Mendes V, Bruyere F, Escoffre JM, Binet A, Lardy H, Marret H, et al. Experience implication in subjective surgical ergonomics comparison between laparoscopic and robot-assisted surgeries. J Robot Surg 2020;14;115-121.

[81] Khandalavala K, Shimon T, Flores L, Armijo PR, Oleynikov D. Emerging surgical robotic technology: a progression toward microbots. Annals of Laparoscopic and Endoscopic Surgery 2019;5.

[82] Gosrisirikul C, Don Chang K, Raheem AA, Rha KH. New era of robotic surgical systems. Asian J Endosc Surg 2018;11;291-299.

[83] Ceylan H, Yasa IC, Kilic U, Hu W, Sitti M. Translational prospects of untethered medical microrobots.

Progress in Biomedical Engineering 2019;1;012002.

[84] Li J, Esteban-Fernandez de Avila B, Gao W, Zhang L, Wang J. Micro/Nanorobots for Biomedicine: Delivery, Surgery, Sensing, and Detoxification. Sci Robot 2017;2.

[85] Sitti M, Ceylan H, Hu W, Giltinan J, Turan M, Yim S, et al. Biomedical Applications of Untethered Mobile Milli/Microrobots. Proc IEEE Inst Electr Electron Eng 2015;103;205-224.

[86] Zemmar A, Lozano AM, Nelson BJ. The rise of robots in surgical environments during COVID-19. Nature Machine Intelligence 2020;2;566-572.

Chapter 5

# Robotic Coronary Artery Bypass Grafting: History, Current Technique, and Future Perspectives

*Ekin Guran, Andrea Amabile and Gianluca Torregrossa*

## Abstract

Coronary Artery Bypass Grafting surgery is the most commonly performed and thoroughly examined adult cardiac surgery procedure in the world. Minimally invasive techniques which include Robotic-Assisted Minimally Invasive Direct Coronary Artery Bypass Grafting and Totally Endoscopic Coronary Artery Bypass Grafting have been helping to lessen the postoperative complications, pain, and length of stay, while enhancing postoperative quality of life of patients. However, practical application of these advanced procedures has yet to be broadly mastered for expanding the usage of minimally invasive robotic assisted techniques. This chapter describes the development and application of Minimally Invasive CABG procedures as well as the current knowledge and future perspectives on Robotic-Assisted CABG procedures.

**Keywords:** coronary artery bypass grafting, minimally invasive coronary artery bypass grafting, robotic-assisted minimally invasive direct coronary artery bypass grafting, totally endoscopic coronary artery bypass grafting, CABG, robotic-assisted CABG, TECAB, minimally invasive CABG, robotic CABG, robotic cardiac surgery

## 1. Introduction

Rapidly developing technologies in the field of surgery have encouraged the shift of conventional techniques towards minimally invasive methods.

Since cardiovascular diseases are the leading cause of death worldwide, causing the greatest threat to public health, it is perfectly reasonable to implement practice with technological advancements to treat cardiovascular diseases with minimally invasive approaches [1].

Robotic-assisted surgery offers the clinical benefits of a minimally invasive approach as well as technical advantages such as enhanced precision and visualization.

Minimally invasive procedures employed in surgical coronary revascularization include Minimally Invasive Direct Coronary Artery Bypass Grafting (MIDCAB), Robotic-Assisted MIDCAB, and Totally Endoscopic Coronary Artery Bypass Grafting (TECAB). MIDCAB is a less invasive method of Coronary Artery Bypass Grafting (CABG), in which the surgical access is obtained by a left anterior



IntechOpen

mini-thoracotomy, instead of a conventional sternotomy. In robotic-assisted MIDCAB, the left internal thoracic artery (LITA) harvest is performed with the robotic platform and is then followed by a direct anastomosis sewn through a small thoracotomy incision. Finally, TECAB is the entirely endoscopic version of the procedure, in which the robotic platform is used for both graft harvesting and coronary anastomosis.

Robotic MIDCAB and TECAB can both be done either on beating heart or on arrested heart, with the aid of cardiopulmonary bypass (CPB) support or not. Whether the operation is conducted on a beating or arrested heart is decided cautiously, considering the vascular status of the patient since the arrested heart approach may provide a better quality of anastomosis. Not only is CPB obligatory on the arrested heart approach, but it also comes in handy on a beating heart approach in patients with poor blood gas exchange, or with multiple vessel disease additionally to badly constructed vascular status [2].

In this chapter, we discuss the currently available robotic-assisted CABG strategies, including Robotic-Assisted MIDCAB, robotic TECAB with the aid of cardiopulmonary bypass (CPB), either on a beating or arrested heart, as well as robotic TECAB without the aid of CPB to achieve single or multivessel coronary grafting performed either with the robotic anastomotic device or in a hand-sewn fashion.,

## 2. History of robotic cardiac surgery

The use of robotic assistance in surgical procedures dates back to 1985, when Kwoh et al. used a robotic system to improve the accuracy of CT-guided brain tumor biopsies [3]. Davies et al. later used robotic techniques for transurethral resection of the prostate in 1991 [4]. Peaked interest in robotic applications in surgery led to the development of new robotic systems. In 1996, Carpentier et al. conducted the first robot-assisted cardiac procedure, which was a mitral valve repair [5]. In 1999, Mohr et al. [6] and Loulmet et al. [7] performed CABG with the aid of a robotic platform. Over time, robotic-assisted CABG procedures evolved from single-vessel to multi-vessel, and its use has since then expanded to the integration with hybrid applications.

## 3. Advantages

### 3.1 Clinical advantages

The shift of conventional procedures towards minimally invasive approaches has allowed patients to benefit from surgical treatment with fewer postoperative complications, reduced morbidity associated with surgical trauma, and shorter length of stay while enhancing the postoperative quality of life and cosmetic outcomes [8].

Robotic-assisted MIDCAB offers a minimally invasive alternative to the traumatic median sternotomy performed in conventional CABG by providing access to the thoracic cavity through a less traumatic left anterior mini-thoracotomy. This approach reduces postoperative pain scores, and also eliminates the usual risk of poor healing following median sternotomy, thus reducing the length of postoperative hospital stay [9, 10].

Sternotomy prolongs the recovery duration and bears the risk of poor healing and deep sternal wound infection (DSWI). Despite the fact that DSWI has a low incidence (between 0.2% and 3%), it is a deadly complication, and it weighs a heavy burden on healthcare with the need of repeated surgical interventions, prolonged length of stay, lower quality of life after CABG surgery, with higher costs [11–13]. Patients with comorbidities such as diabetes mellitus, chronic obstructive pulmonary disease, obesity, peripheral vascular disease have an increased risks of DSWI [14–17] Also, female sex, older age, bilateral internal thoracic artery take-down are independent risk factors on that matter [16–19]. Thanks to its minimally invasive properties, TECAB surgery reduces the risk of DSWI even in BITA take-down surgery [14, 20, 21].

The postoperative overall quality of life is improved in both robotic-assisted CABG and conventional CABG, thanks to enhanced myocardial perfusion obtained by coronary revascularization. Nevertheless, while patients undergoing TECAB achieve this rather rapidly, those undergoing conventional CABG reach the same level of comfort much later due to the greater invasive nature of the sternotomy [22].

In terms of outcomes, robotic-assisted CABG graft patency rates were found to be equivalent to outcomes of the conventional technique [23]. TECAB has yielded excellent results, even in patients with a high risk of mortality [24].

### 3.2 Technical advantages

Robotic-assisted minimally invasive procedures have enabled surgeons to perform surgical procedures with enhanced vision, precision, control, and dexterity [25]. Although the lack of haptic feedback was initially observed as a limitation for robotic surgeons, the Da Vinci system provides outstanding 3D visualization to observe the displacement of tissues which compensates for the lack of tactile feedback [26]. In addition to greatly improved visualization, robotic instrumentation also provides several technical advantages. Built-in motion scaling converts large natural movements to ultraprecise micromovements, and tremor filtration allows smoother and more precise motions of the articulating instrument at the surgical site [27, 28]. The wristed robotic instrumentation and robotic arms provide seven degrees of freedom (three for translation, three for rotation, and one for grasping), rather than only four degrees of movement maintained by the endoscopic devices [29]. Furthermore, robotic-assisted surgery eliminates the "fulcrum effect", otherwise faced by long-shafted endoscopic instruments, in which the hand of the surgeon and the tip of the instrument moves in opposite directions [30].

## 4. Disadvantages

As CABG surgery is the most commonly performed and adult cardiac surgery procedure worldwide, there has been a growing interest in robotic-assisted CABG. However, despite the initial enthusiasm, it did not become as widespread as expected, for reasons such as its steep learning curve, the requirement of an experienced surgical team, and its higher costs [31].

## 5. Patient selection

Each patient should be individually assessed by a multidisciplinary team of cardiac surgeons and cardiologists to determine the best approach regarding myocardial revascularization. Clinical status, associated comorbidities, and anatomical features should be considered when determining the appropriate strategy for myocardial revascularization.

Robotic-assisted CABG is more frequently used to treat total occlusion or ostial stenosis of the left anterior descending (LAD) artery, and occasionally to treat proximal LAD stenosis which is unsuitable for percutaneous intervention. Robotic-assisted CABG is also feasible in the treatment of multivessel disease, though rarely performed, in which both ITAs and a second graft can be used individually or with sequential anastomosis techniques [2].

Minimally invasive CABG may also be integrated with a hybrid approach, i.e., achieving simultaneous or delayed complete revascularization with both CABG (usually for the left coronary system) and percutaneous coronary interventions (PCI) (usually for the right coronary system), providing patients with the advantages of each technique in the least invasive manner possible [32].

Robotic-assisted MIDCAB is one of the most commonly performed robotic-assisted CABG procedures around the globe [33]. This is often conducted off-pump and consists of the endoscopic harvesting of the LITA with robotic instrumentation followed by direct anastomosis of the left anterior descending (LAD) artery through a left anterior mini-thoracotomy. Robotic MIDCAB may be preferred in patients with isolated disease of the LAD, or within the framework of hybrid coronary revascularization (HCR) strategy to treat patients with multivessel coronary stenosis along with PCI to all diseased non-LAD vessels [34]. Although robotic MIDCAB is not optimal for hemodynamically unstable patients, patients with limited pulmonary reserve or patients with significantly impaired left ventricular systolic function, favorable outcomes have been previously reported [35].

Although patient selection for robotic-assisted CABG was initially limited to non-redo patients with isolated single-vessel or double-vessel disease rather than multi-vessel disease and those with preserved ventricular function, inclusion criteria has since then broadened to include also redo patients, provided one internal thoracic artery (ITA) is still adequate for grafting. Studies have demonstrated that the procedure was viable in patients with a history of previous open CABG [36], MIDCAB [33], and TECAB [37].

In current practice, many patients with a confirmed indication for surgical myocardial revascularization can be deemed as candidates for robotic-assisted CABG. Potential contraindications include acute myocardial ischemia, serious multi-organ dysfunction, severe pulmonary dysfunction, restricted workspace inside the thoracic cavity (e.g., in severe pectus excavatum), thoracic adhesions, and obesity (BMI > 35 kg/m2) [38]. Relative contraindications to TECAB are serious left pleural fibrosis in patients with a history of chronic lung disease or lung surgery. Management with an off-pump approach may not be always feasible in patients with severely impaired lung function and peripheral cardiopulmonary bypass (CPB) support to enhance gas exchange may be considered in these cases. Emergent procedures and patients with advanced left ventricular systolic dysfunction potentially requiring advanced postoperative myocardial support are currently ruled out [32].

## 6. Anesthetic approach

Team coordination and communication are fundamental aspects to prevent complications in any surgical operation. This is especially important during robotic-assisted surgery, considering the physical distance between team members. Therefore, we recommend that all team members (consisting of a console surgeon, tableside assistant, anesthesiologist, perfusionist, circulating nurse, and all others who are involved) are equipped with Bluetooth headsets to ensure smooth and effective communication.

To be on par with rapid advancements in the field of robotic surgery, anesthesiologists had to overcome new challenges such as longer surgical times, problems with single-lung ventilation in the presence of coronary artery disease, and enhanced expertise in transesophageal echocardiography (TEE) [39]. Other drawbacks include the higher physical distance from the patient than usual, dealing with a bulky device onto the operative field, managing the specific patient positioning, and maintaining patient immobility while preventing prolonged postoperative recovery time due to the excessive use of neuromuscular blocking agents.

Because of the reasons stated above, robotic-assisted CABG procedures require an experienced cardiothoracic anesthesiologist. The console surgeon, tableside surgeon, and anesthesiologist must all be coordinated and in harmony throughout the entire procedure.

Anesthetic management consists of single-lung ventilation, as well as right radial artery pressure monitoring and central venous catheterization for hemodynamic monitorization throughout the surgery. Single-lung ventilation may be accomplished with either a double-lumen endotracheal tube or a single-lumen endotracheal tube with the usage of a left endobronchial balloon blocker. External defibrillator pads should be located across the heart beforehand, one on the right lateral chest and the other one on the left scapula. Near-infrared spectroscopy (NIRS) is also strongly advised to prevent postoperative cognitive dysfunction [40].

Due to the closed nature of the operation, monitoring TEE throughout the procedure is essential. TEE contributes invaluable information regarding baseline cardiac capacity and may be used to diagnose undetected pathologies. TEE ensures secure and a pinpoint positioning of guidewires and cannula for peripheral cardiopulmonary bypass. TEE is imperative for the management and safety of robotic CABG procedures since it allows for immediate detection of rare but catastrophic complications of peripheral cannulation, including superior vena cava injury or aortic dissection [41].

## 7. Surgical procedure

### 7.1 Patient positioning

Some preliminary steps including patient set up, cardiopulmonary perfusion, placement of the ports, and robotic-assisted harvesting of LITA are in the same manner for both robotic-assisted CABG surgeries. While the MIDCAB procedure continues with de-novo incision after LITA harvesting for making a direct hand-sewn anastomosis between the LITA and the coronary target, the TECAB procedure continues with robotic-assisted coronary anastomosis [31].

After the left lung is deflated, three robotic ports are placed into the left thoracic cavity under direct view. First, the camera port is located in the left fourth intercostal space in the anterior axillary line. The right and left robotic instrument ports are placed under endoscopic visualization in the second and sixth intercostal spaces, respectively, in alignment with the camera port.

The robotic-assisted anastomosis part of the TECAB surgery requires two additional ports which should be placed after robotic ITA harvesting and graft preparation. A 12-mm 4th robotic port is used to insert the Endo-wrist™ stabilizer, placed in the left subcostal space, medial side of the midclavicular line. And finally, to deliver the Cardica Flex A™ anastomotic device, a 15-mm port (Ethicon Surgical, Somerville NJ) is inserted in the 2nd intercostal space on the left midclavicular line.

After the ports placed, the table is lowered and tilted 10° to the right, and the da Vinci Si system (Intuitive Surgical, Sunnyvale, California, United States) is docked with the robotic cart, which is generally located at approximately 60° angle to the table from the right side. This positioning is to decrease the interference between the robotic arms.

Continuous warm humidified CO2 insufflation should be maintained to properly dilate the surgical area and provide sufficient pleural workspace. Intrathoracic pressure must be kept within 8–12 mmHg not to compromise hemodynamic stability. Air insufflation systems should be used at low levels since excessive use of insufflation may cause endothelial damage. We recommend maintaining the CO2 insufflation settings while entering the right thoracic cavity for BITA harvesting. Of note, using two CO2 insufflation is convenient in TECAB surgery to protect the vascular structures and heart itself from injury as a result of a sudden loss of pressure.

### 7.2 Cardiopulmonary perfusion and myocardial protection

Robotic-assisted CABG can be executed either on an arrested or beating heart. Whether the operation will be performed with the arrested or beating heart approach is decided cautiously considering the vascular status of the patient since the arrested heart approach may provide a better quality of anastomosis. CBP support is obligatory in the arrested heart approach. But it is not the only case that requires CBP support. It can be also used in the beating heart approach to improve poor blood gas exchange and in patients with multiple vessel disease additionally to badly constructed vascular status [2].

Considering arrested heart or beating heart surgery in need of hemodynamic or pulmonary support, the peripheral CPB method is usually the chosen one. The CPB support during TECAB is considerably low (less than 2%) and most of which used to improve gas exchange rate during single lung ventilation [31].

Since peripheral CPB support is recommended in case CPB is needed, femoral vessels should be prepared. A transverse left inguinal incision is made above the inguinal ligament to expose the femoral artery and vein. Firstly, a 4–0 polypropylene purse-string suture is implanted in each vessel which is followed by tourniquet application. Then, the introduction of a perfusion cannula with a sidearm (21-F or 23-F) into the femoral artery is underway. At last, cannulation of the femoral vein with a 25-F venous cannula is performed.

IntraClude™ balloon occlusion catheter (Edwards Lifesciences, Irvine, CA, USA) or a mechanical cross-clamp (e. g. Chitwood™, Scanlon International, Minneapolis, MN, USA) with antegrade cardioplegia are the preferred tools to be used during aortic cross-clamping and cardioplegia delivery. Because of the reason that pulmonary artery interposition makes cross-clamping the aorta from the left chest to be technically challenging, balloon occlusion catheter remains to be the preferred one.

TEE guidance is essential during the insertion of the IntraClude™ balloon occlusion catheter towards the aortic root. The balloon should be placed above the sino-tubular junction, and well below the brachiocephalic trunk. Antegrade, cold blood cardioplegia should be administered repeatedly according to the chosen cardioplegia solution.

### 7.3 ITA harvesting

After the endoscopic camera (30-degree up) is inserted, monopolar curved scissors are equipped to the right arm while Maryland bipolar forceps are equipped to the left one. Then dissection and reflection of the pericardial fat pad are performed. Pinpoint determination of the opening site of the pericardium is decided according to the grafting approach, since the pericardiotomy should be performed anterior to the phrenic nerve and towards the apex of the heart for LAD targets, and pericardium should be entered posterior to the phrenic nerve for circumflex marginal coronary targets. In addition, a small-scaled pericardial incision posterior to the phrenic nerve can both help drainage of the pericardial space post-operatively as well as in our belief it helps to prevent postoperative pericarditis. Since the protection of the phrenic nerve is of vital importance, care should always be taken to avoid injury during pericardial manipulation.

After reaching the surface of the epicardium, the angiogram becomes particularly useful to point out the correct coronary targets. Following the description of the targets for endoscopic grafting, attention is directed towards the ITA(s).

The two ITAs are adjacent to each other and to the heart from the endothoracic viewpoint than is commonly appreciated, considering the greater majority of surgeons only encountered them in open CABG procedures when the sternum is widely separated by a midline sternotomy incision. Thereby, either of the ITA can be used as an in-situ conduit to graft the LAD and high marginal branches.

Due to the lack of tactile feedback, excess tension should be avoided, and extra care should be taken to avoid damaging the ITAs. ITA harvesting begins from the proximal side, until its origin from the subclavian artery, to enable it to utilize its entire length. The harvesting is preferably performed as a skeletonized technique by the dissection of the artery from the fascia, intercostal muscles, and the encircling tissues to take maximum advantage of the length of the artery and also to profit from higher flow capacity [42]. This technique also assists in maneuvering the graft within the thoracic cavity and also paves the way for the assessment of the endoscopic transit-time Doppler flow. Despite the advantages of this technique, many surgeons, especially those at an earlier phase of their robotics training, still goes for the ITAs as pedicled grafts.

If the right internal thoracic artery (RITA) is to be used, it should also be the first to be harvested. Otherwise, the left thoracic artery (LITA) should be chosen without the opening of the right pleura. For both conduits, the dissection procedure is identical.

At the beginning of the RITA harvesting procedure, the finest view while dissecting of the substernal anterior mediastinal fibro-fatty tissue and during entry into the right thoracic space is given by a 0-degree robotic endoscope. After the dissection is done, the RITA should be harvested using a 30-degree (focused-up) scope. When instruments are guided into the right pleural space, it is of vital importance to prevent physical contact with the heart. Careful maneuvers should be undertaken in order to position the cameras safely near to the right pleural workspace, and the instruments should first be spotted by a direct vision from the left pleural area and then removed from there.

The endothoracic fascia and the transverse thoracic muscle are divided to uncover the vessel while harvesting RITA. For the monopolar spatula and micro bipolar forceps (20 W), a low electro-cautery setting is used to cauterize narrow vessel branches, while the larger ones should be divided with robotically applied metal clips.

The Endo-Wrist stabilizer is used to compress the anterior mediastinal tissue to optimally harvest the proximal and distal sections of the RITA. This instrument is extremely useful in TECAB surgery to help stabilize the target during the anastomosis, whether it is done on a beating or arrested heart, but it is also practical during a conduit harvesting process since it allows routine BITA harvesting regardless of the anatomical variations between the patients. It is inserted through a 12-mm subcostal 4th robotic port placed between the xiphoid process and the midclavicular line as mentioned before. When docking the fourth robotic arm a "setup joint" adjustment towards cephalic direction is recommended in order to avoid external conflicts between robotic arms.

When executing the mediastinal fat retraction with the Endo-Wrist stabilizer, care must be taken to secure that suited proximal dissection of the RITA is accomplished and adequate conduit length is provided. The 0-degree scope is ideally used to harvest the proximal RITA; the artery should be dissected up till the first intercostal branches are uncovered; then several metal clips should be used to divide the medial right internal thoracic vein. In order to widen the anteroposterior space especially in patients with narrow space between the sternum and the heart and thereby decrease the risk of instrument-induced arrhythmias, the stabilizer is then positioned on the epicardial surface while dissecting the caudal extremity of the RITA. Once the RITA is almost entirely liberated but not distally divided from the encircling tissue, attention is drawn to the LITA, which is harvested likewise as mentioned before.

The conduits are prepared with intraluminal papaverine solution injection after the harvesting of both ITAs from the loose areolar tissue is completed over their total length. A bulldog clamp is placed on the proximal RITA after heparinization. To evaluate sufficient flow through the conduit, the distal end of the RITA was occluded by a metal clip, and partially transected only the proximal site of this clip with the help of robotic Potts scissors afterward. Meanwhile, a syringe of 1:20 diluted papaverine solution connected to a 20-G Perifix® epidural catheter (B. Braun, Melsungen, Germany) is operated by the table-side assistant via the working port and then inserted tenderly by the console surgeon into the lumen of the RITA. Papaverine is injected as the catheter is removed. The table-side assistant should extract arterial blood before infusing the papaverine to confirm the correct intra-luminal catheter location. The catheter should then be slowly retrieved, and immediately after catheter removal, the RITA is distally clipped. For LITA, the same procedure is repeated.

### 7.4 Coronary target(s) preparation

If robotic-assisted MIDCAB surgery is the selected approach, this step continues with removing the robotic instruments and ports and expanding the camera port incision to a 5-cm left anterior mini-thoracotomy to provide direct access to the selected coronary targets, while TECAB surgery continues with robotic assistance in the rest of the procedure thereby does not need a wider thoracotomy incision. The retractors are used in Robotic-assisted MIDCAB to provide a better view similar to regular MIDCAB surgery. A pericardiotomy is performed through thoracotomy incision, which is applied anteromedially in the direction of the apical part of the heart, imitating the orientation of the LAD thus allowing the ITA to enter the pericardial space without any twist or torsion afterward. After the pericardiotomy, the LAD is exposed and can be stabilized with the help of external vacuum-assisted or pressure-assisted systems. After the coronary target preparation is finished, a direct hand-sewn graft-coronary target anastomosis is applied through the thoracotomy incision in MIDCAB surgery.

TECAB surgery, which stands out among all the surgical myocardial revascularization strategies due to its minimally invasive nature, requires two additional ports which should be placed in this stage of the procedure. A 12-mm 4th robotic port for the Endo-wrist™ stabilizer and finally, a 12 mm or 15-mm working port for coronary anastomosis instead of a de-novo thoracotomy incision.

With the help of the Endo-Wrist stabilizer, the coronary target(s) is stabilized and then exposed. Proper exposure is served by using low cautery energy with gentle opening of the overlying epicardium, which in our belief is more beneficial than sharp dissection to obtain better hemostasis in an endoscopic workspace.

The coronary target is then proximally encircled with a silastic snare Saddleloop™ (Quest Medical, Inc., Allen, TX, USA). To limit the possible venous bleeding at the coronary target sites, the silastic snare application is performed before the delivery of systemic heparinization and dividing the conduits. Upon the completion of coronary target preparation, the patient is heparinized with a specific target of activated clotting time (ACT) for each procedure acting as 300 s for MIDCAB and off-pump TECAB, while should be above 420 s for on-pump-TECAB.

### 7.5 Robotic-assisted coronary anastomosis, device-driven fashion

Contrary to robotic-assisted MIDCAB surgery, the coronary target anastomosis part of TECAB surgery is also completed endoscopically. There are two techniques for robotic-assisted anastomosis and applications differ depending on preference. If device-driven anastomosis is to be made, a 15 mm working port is required to insert C-Port Flex A system; on the other hand, if the hand-sewn technique is to be used, a 12 mm working port is required to embed the coronary shunts and sutures (Ethicon Surgical, Somerville, NJ, USA).

A 30-degree scope is used for better visualization. To begin with the device-driven technique, the left and right robotic arms are equipped with Black Diamond forceps. The stabilizer at the 4th port is replaced with a DeBakey forceps and the 15 mm working port is loaded with the Flex A system to perform the automated coronary anastomosis.

The Flex A device is inserted along with its neutral position which points to the diaphragm as the anvil facing heart and cartridge facing sternum and held by the DeBakey forceps. Then it is rotated in a way that now cartridge faces down while the anvil faces the sternum. Later on, the device is moved vertically to a position that faces the camera. In order to inspect and trim encircling tissue, ITA is also oriented and positioned along with the device. The placement of LITA inside the cartridge can now be ready to complete after the 10-mm linear arteriotomy. Following the placement of heels of the arteriotomy to the designated sites on the cartridge by two Black Diamond forceps, tableside assistant lowers the piercer onto the heel clip and fixates the heel of LITA onto the cartridge. During the next step, which is lowering the shield guard, slight bending of the guard can enhance the hood of the anastomosis. Then, both sides of the heel are positioned to the contrary sides of the cartridge to match with staple bays. During this placement, it is of vital importance that each staple bay is correctly matched with LITA tissue and there should be no folds in the LITA after it is properly positioned. In order to achieve this, firstly tableside assistant lowers the right-wing guard. Then, before lowering the left-wing guard, the assistant should also remove the piercer to fixate LITA in the proper place. Lowering both of the wing guards and fixation of LITA to its proper place marks the loading of the conduit so that the device can now be moved back to its neutral position and placed nearby to the target vessel on the pericardium.

The 4th port is loaded with the Endo-Wrist stabilizer once again to stabilize the coronary target. The silastic snare that encircles the coronary target which previously placed before is now tightened and hemodynamic responses and ECG alterations are observed. ST-segment elevations are tolerated since it's not necessarily a proof of ischemia but can be referred to alterations in signal detection because of the physical displacement of the heart unless followed with hemodynamic compromise. Ischemic preconditioning might be beneficial to prepare the myocardium before coronary occlusion [43].

After the coronary flow is blocked by tightening the silastic snare, a small coronary arteriotomy in the core of a previously placed CV-8 Gore-Tex suture (Gore Medical, Flagstaff, Ariz) is performed by an endo-knife (Snap-Fit; Intuitive

Surgical, Sunnyvale, Calif) using a purse-string stitch. This stitch is required to seal the insertion site of the anvil after the device is removed, since it is not part of the anastomosis. The anvil is then inserted and positioned parallelly to the coronary target. Placement of anvil inside the lumen of the vessel is crucial before moving on with the following steps of the anastomotic procedure. Then, tableside assistant activates the device and performs the anastomosis. Following the proper formation of anastomosis, the cartridge is released, the shield guard is raised, and anvil is discharged.

After the suture is tied, one should always look for potential bleeding. If that's the case, the surgeon should add additional stitches.

Occasional examination of the transit-time flow measurement (TTFM) of the graft is necessary [44–46]. In order to do this, a flexible probe through the port like Medistim (Medistim Inc., Oslo, Norway) can be used. This system provides valuable information about the procedure like mean blood flow, pulsatility index, and percentage diastolic filling. In addition, consideration of the competitive flow should also be closely examined.

If sequential grafting is needed, instead of Flex A device which is only applicable for end-to-side anastomosis, a hand-sewn technique comes into play. Thus, sequential grafting should start with the anastomotic device, then should continue with the hand-sewn approach.

## 7.6 Robotic-assisted, hand-sewn coronary anastomosis

Because of the aforementioned cases, in order to perform robotic-assisted coronary anastomosis, the anastomotic device is not mandatory since the hand-sewn technique is also capable of doing the same procedure.

Histological studies also prove that device-driven anastomosis can be comparable with the hand-sewn anastomosis [47–49].

It is crucial to prepare the anastomotic sites before insertion of the suture in the thoracic cavity with the endo-wrist stabilizer. In order to perform LAD anastomosis, a 30-degree down scope provides better visualization, whereas a 30-degree up (or 0-degree) scope is preferred for left circumflex branch anastomosis. Also, observing some crucial parameters like ECG alterations, variables derived from TEE, and hemodynamic responses during the 5 to 8 minutes of myocardial ischemic preconditioning is recommended. During this period, required items like shunts and sutures can be inserted into the thoracic cavity. After clamping the ITA with a small bulldog clamp, Pott scissors are used to transcend and trim to the adequate length. It is advantageous to clip the distal side of the ITA to the encircling pericardium to deal with the conduit when conducting the anastomosis. Endo-knife (Snap-Fit; Intuitive Surgical, Sunnyvale, California, U.S.) assisted arteriotomy is performed and extended with Pott scissors after a short reperfusion duration.

Both robotic arms are now equipped with Black Diamond forceps. A correct size shunt is now positioned (via the regular off-pump coronary artery bypass techniques) and the snare is released. A double-arm 7–0 Pronova suture is used to induce anastomosis in a continuous manner (Johnson & Johnson Medical, New Brunswick, New Jersey, United States). Suturing from the farthest side of the surgeon is introduced in the center of the arteriotomy, and should be completed on the adjacent side of the surgeon.

The stitches are normally carried out on the coronary artery in an outside-in fashion, but this procedure can be altered in the opposite direction only if there is the presence of calcified plaques within the coronary target wall. The graft is then parachuted onto the target artery. It is advised to insert a shunt within the conduit if there is confusion about the visualization of the heel of the conduit. The suture should be tightened in order to stop bleeding after the suture is finished. The shunt(s) should be withdrawn just before the suture is tightened.

Finally, the proximal snare and the bulldog clamp are released. After performing every anastomosis, TTFM should be evaluated with a flexible MediStim probe. If the pulsatility index is greater than 5 and the mean arterial blood flow is less than 15 mL/min, we recommend that the graft be checked.

### 7.7 Final surgical maneuvers

After the grafting procedures have been finalized with satisfactory results and adequate hemostasis, all the items used in the surgical procedure are cleared away from the thoracic cavity. Extra-pericardial fat that has been transferred to the lateral side is now sutured back to the medial border of the pericardium to cover the anterior face of the heart and the graft, and a 4–0 V-Loc suture (Medtronic, Minneapolis, Minnesota, United States) is used to conduct both of these procedures. The left lung is suctioned in and the lung is reinflated.

A 24-French Blake Drain (Ethicon Inc., Somerville, New Jersey, United States) is placed in the right thoracic cavity through the sub-costal port, and the second 24-French Blake Drain is also placed in the left thoracic cavity through the left port. The robot is undocked, and all the ports are removed.

If the surgery is performed on an arrested heart with CPB support, a 'hot shot' of cardioplegia or warmblood is administered before deflating the endoballoon. Only after the robot is undocked, all ports are removed, and ventilation is fully restored, will separation from the CPB support, protamine administration, and decannulation be carried out. To minimize the risk of bleeding on the port sides, it is strongly recommended to re-inspect the port sides with the scope after protamine is administered. For off-pump TECAB, this is extremely unlikely.

Finally, all port incisions are sealed with subcuticular stitches and in this way, the surgery is now completed.

## 8. Conclusion

At first, the TECAB technique was limited to treating single vessel disease with LITA-LAD anastomosis on an arrested heart with CPB support and in time it is proven to be safe and feasible [50, 51]. Since robotic surgical technology continues its exponential growth, the advancements in the next generations of the da Vinci robotic systems will be expected to enhance treatment options even for the high-risk patients with multivessel disease.

Robotic-assisted, totally endoscopic, off-pump CABG has been shown to be safe and feasible in treating the multivessel disease and offers outstanding results in experienced hands. To achieve successful results, the whole surgical team should master robotic surgery, and be in harmony during the procedure and in the meantime, the highest attention should be directed to the hemodynamic and hemostatic parameters of the patient.

However, the surgeons should note that robotic-assisted CABG surgery has a steep learning curve and should start with gaining experience in the treatment of single-vessel cases before progressing to multivessel procedures. Intensive training on hand-sewn suturing techniques using dry and wet-lab models is essential and highly recommended. Due to the steep learning curve and the lack of excellence centers focused on the robotic-assisted CABG, the interest from the industry has been half-hearted.

Finally, since robotic surgical technology is experiencing exponential growth and expanding its use in many specialties, it is of vital importance for us, the surgeons, to be a part of these advancements and train the next generation of surgeons accordingly in order to help them serve our society with latest minimally invasive approaches.

## Author details

Ekin Guran[1*], Andrea Amabile[2] and Gianluca Torregrossa[3]

1 University of Health Sciences, Ankara, Turkey

2 Yale University, New Haven, Connecticut, USA

3 Main Line Health, Philadelphia, Pennsylvania, USA

*Address all correspondence to: drekinguran@gmail.com

## References

[1] Prevention, C.f.D.C.a. *Underlying Cause of Death, 1999-2019*. 1999-2019 [cited 2021 January 27]; Available from: https://wonder.cdc.gov/ucd-icd10.html.

[2] Onan, B., *Coronary revascularization in robotic cardiac surgery*. Cardiovasc Surg Int, 2018. **5**(1): p. 48-59.

[3] Kwoh, Y.S., et al., *A robot with improved absolute positioning accuracy for CT guided stereotactic brain surgery*. 1988. p. 153-160.

[4] Davies, B., et al., *The development of a surgeon robot for prostatectomies*. Proceedings of the Institution of Mechanical Engineers, Part H: Journal of Engineering in Medicine, 1991. **205**(1): p. 35-38.

[5] Carpentier, A., et al., *Computer assisted open heart surgery. First case operated on with success*. Comptes rendus de l'Academie des sciences. Serie III, Sciences de la vie, 1998. **321**(5): p. 437-442.

[6] Mohr, F.W., et al., *Computer-enhanced coronary artery bypass surgery*. The Journal of thoracic and cardiovascular surgery, 1999. **117**(6): p. 1212-1214.

[7] Loulmet, D., et al., *Endoscopic coronary artery bypass grafting with the aid of robotic assisted instruments*. The journal of thoracic and cardiovascular surgery, 1999. **118**(1): p. 4-10.

[8] Mack, M.J., *Minimally invasive and robotic surgery*. Jama, 2001. **285**(5): p. 568-572.

[9] Yanagawa, F., et al., *Critical Outcomes in Nonrobotic vs Robotic-Assisted Cardiac Surgery*. JAMA Surgery, 2015. **150**(8): p. 771-777.

[10] Jones, B., P. Desai, and R. Poston. *Establishing the case for minimally invasive, robotic-assisted CABG in the treatment of multivessel coronary artery disease*. in *The heart surgery forum*. 2009. NIH Public Access.

[11] Schimmer, C., et al., *Management of poststernotomy mediastinitis: experience and results of different therapy modalities*. Thoracic and Cardiovascular Surgeon, 2008. **56**(4): p. 200-204.

[12] Softah, A., et al., *Wound infection in cardiac surgery*. Annals of Saudi Medicine, 2002. **22**(1-2): p. 105-107.

[13] Graf, K., et al., *Economic aspects of deep sternal wound infections*. European Journal of Cardio-Thoracic Surgery, 2010. **37**(4): p. 893-896.

[14] Phoon, P.H.Y. and N.C. Hwang, *Deep sternal wound infection: diagnosis, treatment and prevention*. Journal of cardiothoracic and vascular anesthesia, 2019.

[15] Omran, A.S., et al., *Superficial and deep sternal wound infection after more than 9000 coronary artery bypass graft (CABG): incidence, risk factors and mortality*. BMC infectious diseases, 2007. **7**(1): p. 1-5.

[16] Grossi, E.A., et al., *Sternal wound infections and use of internal mammary artery grafts*. The Journal of thoracic and cardiovascular surgery, 1991. **102**(3): p. 342-347.

[17] Lillenfeld, D.E., et al., *Obesity and diabetes as risk factors for postoperative wound infections after cardiac surgery*. American journal of infection control, 1988. **16**(1): p. 3-6.

[18] Stahle, E., et al., *Sternal wound complications--incidence, microbiology and risk factors*. European journal of cardio-thoracic surgery, 1997. **11**(6): p. 1146-1153.

[19] Meszaros, K., et al., *Risk factors for sternal wound infection after open heart*

*operations vary according to type of operation.* The Annals of thoracic surgery, 2016. **101**(4): p. 1418-1425.

[20] Benedetto, U., et al., *The influence of bilateral internal mammary arteries on short-and long-term outcomes: a propensity score matching in accordance with current recommendations.* The Journal of thoracic and cardiovascular surgery, 2014. **148**(6): p. 2699-2705.

[21] Gąsior, M., et al., *Hybrid revascularization for multivessel coronary artery disease.* JACC: Cardiovascular Interventions, 2014. **7**(11): p. 1277-1283.

[22] Bonaros, N., et al., *Quality of life improvement after robotically assisted coronary artery bypass grafting.* Cardiology, 2009. **114**(1): p. 59-66.

[23] Kitahara, H., S. Nisivaco, and H.H. Balkhy, *Graft patency after robotically assisted coronary artery bypass surgery.* Innovations, 2019. **14**(2): p. 117-123.

[24] Balkhy, H.H., et al., *Robotic beating heart totally endoscopic coronary artery bypass in higher-risk patients: can it be done safely?* Innovations, 2018. **13**(2): p. 108-113.

[25] Wang, S., J. Zhou, and J. Cai, *Traditional coronary artery bypass graft versus totally endoscopic coronary artery bypass graft or robot-assisted coronary artery bypass graft—meta-analysis of 16 studies.* Eur Rev Med Pharmacol Sci, 2014. **18**(6): p. 790-797.

[26] Meccariello, G., et al., *An experimental study about haptic feedback in robotic surgery: may visual feedback substitute tactile feedback?* Journal of robotic surgery, 2016. **10**(1): p. 57-61.

[27] Prasad, S.M., et al., *Surgical robotics: impact of motion scaling on task performance.* Journal of the American College of Surgeons, 2004. **199**(6): p. 863-868.

[28] Leddy, L.S., T.S. Lendvay, and R.M. Satava, *Robotic surgery: applications and cost effectiveness.* Open Access Surgery, 2010. **3**: p. 99-107.

[29] Chitwood Jr, W.R., et al., *Robotic mitral valve repair: trapezoidal resection and prosthetic annuloplasty with the da Vinci surgical system.* The Journal of thoracic and cardiovascular surgery, 2000. **120**(6): p. 1171-1172.

[30] Dasgupta, P., A. Jones, and I.S. Gill, *Robotic urological surgery: a perspective.* BJU international, 2005. **95**(1): p. 20-23.

[31] Amabile, A., G. Torregrossa, and H.H. Balkhy, *Robotic-assisted coronary artery bypass grafting: current knowledge and future perspectives.* Minerva Cardioangiologica, 2020. **68**(5): p. 497-510.

[32] Ishikawa, N. and G. Watanabe, *Robot-assisted cardiac surgery.* Annals of Thoracic and Cardiovascular Surgery, 2015. **21**(4): p. 322-328.

[33] Balacumaraswami, L., et al., *Minimally invasive direct coronary artery bypass as a primary strategy for reoperative myocardial revascularization.* Innovations, 2010. **5**(1): p. 22-27.

[34] Hemli, J.M. and N.C. Patel, *Robotic cardiac surgery.* Surgical Clinics, 2020. **100**(2): p. 219-236.

[35] Gorki, H., et al., *Long-term survival after minimal invasive direct coronary artery bypass (MIDCAB) surgery in patients with low ejection fraction.* Innovations, 2010. **5**(6): p. 400-406.

[36] Kitahara, H., B. Wehman, and H.H. Balkhy, *Can robotic-assisted surgery overcome the risk of mortality in cardiac reoperation?* Innovations, 2018. **13**(6): p. 438-444.

[37] Nisivaco, S., et al., *Redo robotic endoscopic beating heart coronary bypass (TECAB) after previous TECAB.* The Annals of thoracic surgery, 2017. **104**(6): p. e417-e419.

[38] Bonatti, J., et al., *Robotic totally endoscopic coronary artery bypass grafting: current status and future prospects*. Expert review of medical devices, 2020. **17**(1): p. 33-40.

[39] Chauhan, S. and S. Sukesan, *Anesthesia for robotic cardiac surgery: an amalgam of technology and skill*. Annals of cardiac anaesthesia, 2010. **13**(2): p. 169.

[40] Ortega-Loubon, C., et al., *Near-infrared spectroscopy monitoring in cardiac and noncardiac surgery: pairwise and network meta-analyses*. Journal of clinical medicine, 2019. **8**(12): p. 2208.

[41] Bernstein, W.K. and A. Walker, *Anesthetic issues for robotic cardiac surgery*. Annals of cardiac anaesthesia, 2015. **18**(1): p. 58.

[42] Wendler, O., et al., *Free flow capacity of skeletonized versus pedicled internal thoracic artery grafts in coronary artery bypass grafts*. European journal of cardio-thoracic surgery, 1999. **15**(3): p. 247-250.

[43] Balkhy, H.H., et al., *Integrating coronary anastomotic connectors and robotics toward a totally endoscopic beating heart approach: review of 120 cases*. The Annals of thoracic surgery, 2011. **92**(3): p. 821-827.

[44] Neumann, F.-J., et al., *2018 ESC/EACTS Guidelines on myocardial revascularization*. European heart journal, 2019. **40**(2): p. 87-165.

[45] Kieser, T.M., et al., *Transit-time flow predicts outcomes in coronary artery bypass graft patients: a series of 1000 consecutive arterial grafts*. European journal of cardio-thoracic surgery, 2010. **38**(2): p. 155-162.

[46] Mujanović, E., E. Kabil, and J. Bergsland, *Transit time flowmetry in coronary surgery-an important tool in graft verification*. Bosnian journal of basic medical sciences, 2007. **7**(3): p. 275.

[47] Balkhy, H.H., et al., *The C-Port distal coronary anastomotic device is comparable with a hand-sewn anastomosis: human histological case study*. Innovations, 2018. **13**(2): p. 140-143.

[48] Balkhy, H.H., et al., *Multicenter assessment of grafts in coronaries: midterm evaluation of the C-Port Device (The MAGIC Study)*. Innovations, 2018. **13**(4): p. 273-281.

[49] Hashimoto, M., T. Ota, and H. Balkhy, *Robotic off-pump totally endoscopic hand-sewn coronary artery bypass using in-situ bilateral internal mammary artery*. Multimedia manual of cardiothoracic surgery: MMCTS, 2020. **2020**.

[50] De Cannière, D., et al., *Feasibility, safety, and efficacy of totally endoscopic coronary artery bypass grafting: multicenter European experience*. The Journal of thoracic and cardiovascular surgery, 2007. **134**(3): p. 710-716.

[51] Argenziano, M., et al., *Results of the prospective multicenter trial of robotically assisted totally endoscopic coronary artery bypass grafting*. The Annals of thoracic surgery, 2006. **81**(5): p. 1666-1675.

Section 3

# Robotic Assisted Surgery B

Chapter 6

# Catheter Robots in the Cardiovascular System

*Marton Berczeli, Peter Legeza and Alan Lumsden*

## Abstract

Robotic-assisted endovascular therapy is a novel approach to augment precise skill requirements while simultaneously reducing radiation exposure. The CorPath system enhances the scope of minimally invasive procedures and facilitates the interventionalists to perform procedures in the field of vascular surgery, neurosurgery and interventional cardiology. The reason for increasing interest in the CorPath system is the ability to control these robots through wireless connection, raising the possibility for remote interventions. CorPath is currently the only commercially available endovascular robotic system. Robotic-assisted approach has a high technical success rate in the field of peripheral vascular and coronary interventions and has encouraging results regarding neurointerventions. Remote endovascular procedures may transform the future of stroke treatment in areas where distance-related time loss can affect procedural outcome.

**Keywords:** Robotic-surgery, endovascular robotics, radiation protection, CorPath system, remote surgery, tele-robotic

## 1. Introduction

Our group has a long-standing interest in catheter robotics. This began with the initial launch of Hansen robotic platform for left atrial ablation then followed the evolution of the Hansen system for peripheral interventions [1, 2]. These early studies clearly demonstrated the feasibility of navigating inside the vascular system safely and effectively and outlined some of the future directions for robotic catheter evolution: integrating into imaging, remote control, fluoro-less navigation using electromagnetic fields and autonomous movement [3]. The development of endovascular robotic catheters was seriously interrupted, when Hansen was acquired Auris, who recognized the importance of being able to navigate robotically through long thin tubes, in their case, bronchi. One real challenge of these high-tech start-up companies is the prodigious amount of capital required to develop these technologies. The Auris endobronchial navigation platform (Monarch, Auris Health Inc., Redwood, CA, USA) recently acquired by Johnson & Johnson (New Brunswick, NJ, USA) for 4 billion dollars emphasizes the promise and value which this technology can bring to the clinical area. Currently the only endovascular robot available is from Corindus (Corindus, Siemens-Healthineers Company, Waltham, MA, USA). This will therefore be extensively described in the manuscript. Corindus was recently acquired by Siemens (Siemens-Healthineers, Erlangen, Germany), heralding the real possibility that "preflight" of a robot integrated into a fused image may at last move from fantasy to reality.

## 2. Robotic assistance and radiation protection

The demand for minimally invasive procedures is rapidly increasing. In an endovascular era, the radiation exposure is a crucial factor while performing these procedures on a day-by-day basis. There are several techniques currently available to reduce radiation, but robotic-assisted procedures are considered a different approach. The technique's advantage is that the operator does not have to be next to the patient [4]. The operator can sit behind radiation-shielded platform or away from the operating room by wireless connection (**Figure 1**) without the need of wearing a lead apron [6]. The greatest reduction of radiation is therefore on the primary physician, but the assistants can also keep more distance from the radiation source receiving smaller amount of dose levels [7].

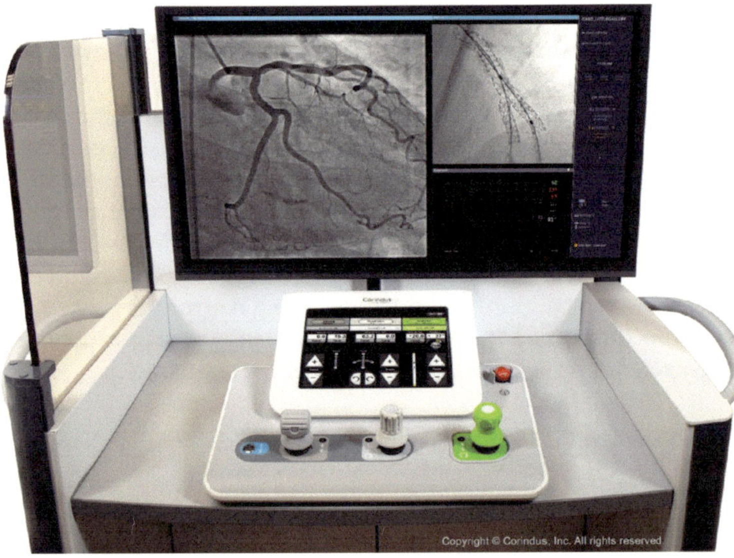


**Figure 1.**
*Robotic console workstation with radiation shielding. The monitors show live fluoroscopy images and patient vitals (© Corindus Inc., used with permission) [5].*

## 3. Robotic systems

**Table 1** demonstrates characteristics of the below presented endovascular robotic systems (**Table 1**).

### 3.1 Magellan system

The first endovascular robotic system was the Magellan Robotic Catheter system (Hansen Medical, Mountain View, California, USA). It was designed for cardiac ablations. It consists a remote wire and catheter manipulator with two available steerable catheter systems. One with a 6 Fr inner leader catheter with a 180-degree multidirectional articulation and a 9 Fr outer sheath with a 90-degree multidirectional manipulation. The other is a 6 Fr low-profile system with two bending sections created for navigating in smaller vessels. The manipulation is done with different tightening of wires integrated into the catheters. The manipulator is mounted on the operating table and allows advancement, retraction, catheter

| Robotic system | Compatible wires | Compatible catheters | Therapeutic device delivery | Navigation | Remote capability |
|---|---|---|---|---|---|
| Magellan | 0.014, 0.018, 0.035 | 6 Fr or 9 Fr Magellan Robotic catheter system | Robotically stabilized manual delivery | Wire and catheter advancement-retraction; 6Fr catheter 180° multidirectional angulation; 9Fr catheter 90° multidirectional angulation | No |
| CorPath 200 | 0.014 | Any commercially available 5–7 Fr catheter | Robotic Rx device delivery | Rx-device advancement, retraction; Wire advancement retraction, rotation | Yes |
| CorPath GRX | 0.014 | Any commercially available 5–7 Fr catheter | Robotic Rx device delivery | Rx-device advancement, retraction; Wire advancement retraction, rotation; Guide-catheter advancement retraction, rotation | Yes |

**Table 1.**
*Technical summary of endovascular robotic systems.*

bending and rotation of the system also. The control panel is located outside of the operating room. It had a console and monitors to show the real-time fluoroscopic images and the catheter orientation as well. The disadvantage of the system is that the therapeutic devices cannot be delivered remotely it has to be done manually with robotic support. The system is approved by the FDA and CE marked, but it is not widely adopted and also not available commercially [8], later the technology was acquired by Auris Health Inc.

### 3.2 CorPath 200

The CorPath 200 robotic system is an endovascular, remotely guided system primarily developed for percutaneous coronary intervention purposes. The first publication appeared in 2011 using it for a coronary angioplasty. The system has two major components: a bedside unit and the interventional cockpit. The cockpit is a mobile radiation-shielded station to perform the intervention. It has two joysticks for device manipulation and monitors for real-time information about the patient's vitals and the actual procedural field (fluoroscopic and subtracted images). This allows an operator to perform an intervention remotely from the cockpit. The robotic arm is mounted to the table and contains the robotic drive and the attached single-use cassette (**Figure 2**). The arm is flexible, so an optimal angle positioning to the access site is achievable. The single-use cassette holds the wire, stent or balloon if loaded into the system and it is connected to a guiding catheter. In order to establish a stable connection with the guide catheter, it has a support track that prevents bending or bleeding while manipulating with the catheter. The cockpit and the robotic drive are connected via communication cables. The system is compatible with 0.014-inch guidewires, rapid exchange (RX) catheter, balloon

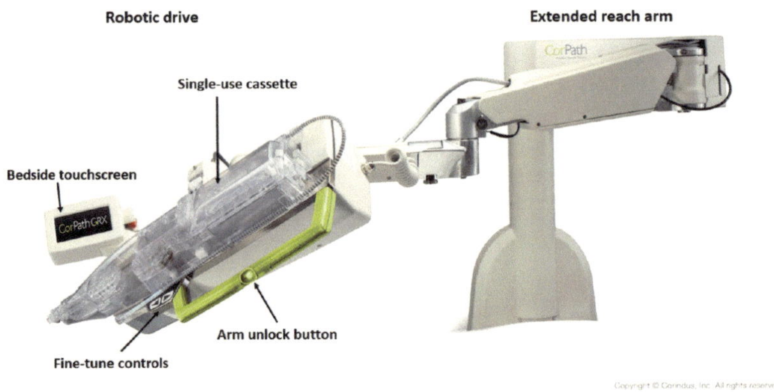


**Figure 2.**
*The CorPath system's robotic arm loaded with a single-use cassette. The whole set-up is mounted to the surgical table (© Corindus Inc., used with permission) [5].*

and stent systems. Additional feature is to measure lesion length by passing the balloon through it then retracting it. The advance and retract functions operate with a 1 mm increment. Through the joysticks the operator can manipulate with the wire and the rapid exchange devices, but the guide catheter control is not available in the CorPath 200. Therefore, a target vessel has to be approached manually. For the wire rotate, advance and retract functions are available, but for the RX devices rotate is not.

### 3.3 CorPath GRX

The next generation Corindus robotic system is the GRX. The major advantage is that it includes an active control on a guide catheter. Thus, the catheter has similar features as a wire in the CorPath 200 system, which is advance retract and rotate. This addition involves an extra joystick inserted into the control panel (**Figure 3**). The extent of guide catheter remote movement is 20 cm, therefor the target lesion has to be approached manually by the operator, but crossing the lesion and device delivery can be completed with the robot.

Another feature is the bedside touchscreen on the robotic drive that allows device exchange. This generation of CorPath robots have a turbo button which facilitates faster device movement and also a rotate-on-retract (RoR) function [9, 10]. RoR if turned on is an automated movement of the wire that provides a 270-degree rotation of the wire every time its retracted, which facilitates target vessel/side-branch cannulation mimicking manual rotation of the guidewire.

The newest features of the GRX are the wiggle, spin and dotter options. All of these were implemented based on experts' different lesion crossing techniques. The wiggle oscillates the guidewire upon advance to prevent prolapse in tortuous anatomy. The spin utilizes clockwise and counterclockwise rotation of the guide-wire, while the dotter can be used for narrow or calcified lesions based on its small, rapid back-and-forth movements during advance.

Every generation of Corindus robotics are platform independent, which means that they are compatible with every type of operating room or catheter lab suite. The robotic drive is draped to preserve sterility in an approximately 2 minutes. The GRX system has FDA approval and CE marked, currently available to use for percutaneous coronary angioplasties and peripheral vascular interventions. It is commercially available and costs in between 500 and 650 000 USD, plus additional single-use cassette and device costs [11].

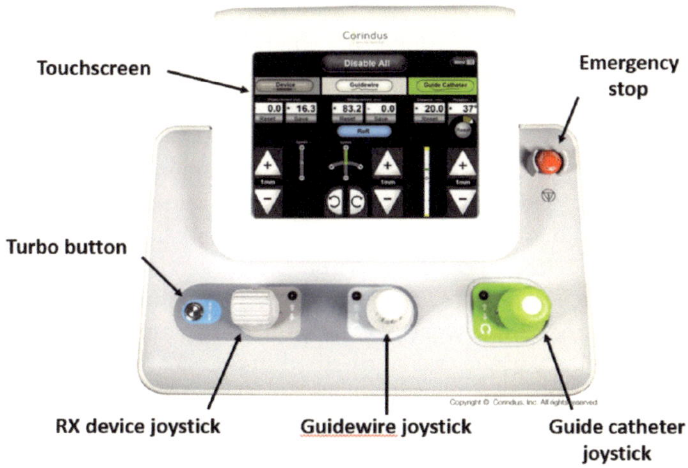


**Figure 3.**
*The new console panel of the GRX system. The three joysticks control the wire, guide catheter and the stent/ balloon. The panel consist a touchscreen that also allows manipulation of the devices (© Corindus Inc., used with permission) [5].*

## 4. Clinical experience

### 4.1 Percutaneous coronary interventions

The first-in-human study regarding coronary angioplasty was published in 2011. Granada and colleagues reported 8 patients, who underwent PCI with the CorPath 200 system. Their data showed a 97% decrease in radiation exposure to the operator with a 97.9% procedural success rate [4]. The first multicenter study with robotic-assisted coronary interventions was the PRECISE study (percutaneous robotically-enhanced coronary intervention) [12]. The study was conducted with the CorPath 200 system and enrolled 164 patients with simple coronary lesions. The inclusion criteria were coronary artery stenosis above 50%, with the diameter in between 2.5–4 mm and with a length that could be covered by one stent. This prospective trial reported a 95.2% decrease in radiation level and a 97.6% success rate. The improvement of the newer generation devices allowed a wider potential application for the robotic assisted therapy as well. The CORA-PCI (Complex Robotically Assisted Percutaneous Coronary Intervention) trial focused on patients with complex coronary artery lesions. Patients were treated by a single operator and a total of 334 PCI-s were analyzed [13]. The results reported a 91.7% technical success and a 99.1% clinical success with robotic-assisted PCI. The study showed that the approach is a viable alternative to manually conducted PCI-s. Regarding postintervention outcomes [14] Walters and colleagues reported non-inferior results in major adverse (cardiac) events at 6 and 12 months also [15]. In 2020, Patel et all. Published their data showing a significant reduction in radiation exposure to patients and medical staff also [16].

### 4.2 Peripheral vascular interventions

The first-in-man study evaluating efficacy of robotic-assisted peripheral arterial lesion cannulation was a prospective, single-armed study by Bismuth et al. [17]. The trial focused on navigating successfully and safely through lesions ranging from simple to complex. The results showed a 100% successful navigation rate and 19 of the 20 lesions were able to be treated by robotic-assisted means using the Magellan system. This study concluded that the robotic-assisted cannulation and treatment are feasible options even for complex peripheral arterial lesions. **Table 2** summarizes the clinical studies completed with the CorPath 200 system (**Table 2**).

The RAPID (Robotic-Assisted Peripheral Intervention for peripheral arterial Disease) trial was a single-arm prospective non-randomized study with symptomatic PAD patients [18]. The inclusion criteria were life-limiting femoro-popliteal stenoses above 50% or occlusion. Total of 20 patients with 29 lesions were treated, primary endpoints were technical success and safety, secondary endpoints included clinical procedural success, fluoroscopy time, contrast volume, procedure time, and adverse events. The procedures were performed from an antegrade femoral punctures, balloon angioplasty alone was performed in 65.5% and in the rest of the cases manually deployed stenting was required. The study reported 100% technical and clinical success without any significant major adverse event. The study's secondary outcome also demonstrated a reduced fluoroscopy time compared to studies treating similar lesions in a conventional manner. These favourable results provided the CorPath system F.D.A. approval for peripheral vascular interventions.

In 2020, the results of the RAPID II trial were published. This study focused on robotic-assisted drug-eluting balloon deployment in the peripheral vascular system [19]. The data of 20 patients reported technical success in all cases, without any major adverse events associated with the device.

The robotic system was used in the below the knee region also. Successful treatments were presented in the posterior tibial artery, tibio-peroneal trunk and in the proximal peroneal artery also [20].

A case-series of robotic-assisted percutaneous renal artery stenting has also been published with promising results and no major adverse events reported [21, 22].

### 4.3 Endovascular aneurysm repair (EVAR) and robotic assistance

Complex aneurysm treatments are technically challenging and more time consuming, therefore both the patient and the medical staff are exposed to higher radiation. The optimistic results from robotic-assisted target lesion/vessel cannulations pioneered the use of the system in endovascular aneurysm repairs also [23]. A feasibility study on an aortic model with the Magellan system showed lesser cannulation time, reduced radiation exposure and reduced number of catheter movements [24]. They highlighted also that with the assistance of the robot to overcome complex cannulations it is not necessarily required to have a well-experienced operator. In another arch model they concluded that robotic

| Clinical trial | Year of publication | Intervention | Treated lesions | Technical success rate (%) | Clinical success rates (%) |
|---|---|---|---|---|---|
| Peripheral vascular | | | | | |
| RAPID [18] | 2016 | R-PVI | 20 | 100 | 100 |
| RAPID II [19] | 2018 | R-PVI | 24 | 100 | 100 |
| Coronary | | | | | |
| PRECISE [12] | 2013 | R-PCI | 164 | 97.6 | 98.8 |
| CORA-PCI [13] | 2016 | R-PCI | 157 | 91.7 | 99.1 |
| REMOTE PCI [16] | 2017 | Tele-PCI | 22 | 86.4 | N/A |

**Table 2.**
*Robotic-assisted clinical studies.*

assistance reduced vessel wall contact and reduced navigational time [25]. More precise navigation was seen in human subjects as well. Comparing conventional and robotic catheter placement and retraction in patients undergoing TEVAR [26]. They recorded a significantly reduced cerebral embolization with the system, which was associated with the lesser number of catheter-vessel wall contacts during the procedure. There is no data currently available with the use of Corindus robotics in EVAR.

### 4.4 Carotid and neurointerventions

Robotic-assisted carotid artery stenting is the boundary of peripheral and neurointerventions. A recently published prospective feasibility study enrolled 13 patients who underwent this procedure. They reported technical success in all of the 13 cases, without postoperative neurological complications using the Magellan system [27].

The CorPath system underwent several modifications to become applicable in the field of neurointerventions. One of these modifications is the additional Y-adapter that enables the use of additional microcatheters, another modification is the active device fixation, which allows the operator to maintain guidewire position during catheter movements. Active guide catheter control also supports vessel cannulation [28]. A preclinical feasibility study on a porcine model was conducted to prove safe robotic navigation in neurovasculature sized vessels of the pig [29]. Based on this trial the use of the CorPath GRX system was authorized in New-Zealand, Australia and the European Union. Although the first-in-human use of the robotic system happened in Canada, when a basilar aneurysm was treated with robotic support [30]. Britz et al. used the GRX system to treat arterio-venous malformation by embolization in a pig model [31].

### 4.5 Robotic-assisted remote interventions

The upgrade on the CorPath system allowed the GRX model to be controlled remotely. Hence tele-stenting become a possible treatment option and a new aspect of robotic-assisted therapies become available. This approach does not require the operator to be in the operating room or next to the patient, the whole system is capable of being controlled from another hospital or office through telecommunication. The setup is provided by local area network and the two sites are using telepresence systems. This includes patient's vital parameters, live or stored fluoroscopy data displayed on monitors and an additional monitor with an overall view of the suite. Communication between the medical staff can be enhanced through wireless headsets [32]. There are multiple studies discussing the safety and feasibility of remote PCI [33–35]. Key factors of the procedure are the network stability and the communication of the medical team. Studies on simulators and on in-vivo models focusing on network latency reported that signal transmission should be below 250 ms not to influence the procedure outcome. The tele-stenting involved five in-human PCIs with a 53 ms mean command delay from a 20 miles distance [36].

## 5. Limitation of the CorPath system

Currently both the CorPath 200 and the GRX model are only compatible with 0.014-inch wires and rapid exchange delivery systems. The upcoming generations of the CorPath systems will be able to manipulate 0.035-inch wires also, which will provide better support for more challenging procedures and could broaden the area of robotic-assisted procedures.

Results of robotic-assisted peripheral vascular interventions have been presented in several regions, but the utility of this approach remains unclear in complex and different scenarios such as chronic total occlusions, severely calcified lesions or obliterative diseases affecting bifurcations. Currently there is no data available in the use of mesenteric or celiac interventions and also the system was not yet used for EVAR. Although there is a demand to perform parts of complex aneurysm procedures to reduce radiation exposure and to reduce manipulation and the number of wire-vessel wall contacts. Active control of the guiding catheters may provide a possible solution to this problem [31].

It is important to emphasize that the published trials and studies reported excellent outcomes and good intravascular navigation, the absence of haptic feedbacks may have an effect on procedural outcomes [23]. This could be an important factor, when maneuvering in smaller vessels like coronary, cerebral and visceral vessels. For this reason, the precise control over the endovascular devices is mandatory and a crucial factor of procedural success [5].

## 6. Future prospects

Robot-assisted endovascular therapy has its benefits and limitations, but it is relatively a new option in the armamentarium of endovascular specialists. The persistent improvements and expanding indication fields provide a faster evolution and modifications of the toolset used for endovascular procedures. Many of these new techniques might not be implemented into robotic-assisted interventions, but basic procedures like vessel cannulation, angioplasty, stenting, angiography or coil delivery become possible to accomplish by robotic assistance.

The advancement of robotic techniques could provide better intravascular navigation and result in significant radiation time decrease for procedures requiring advanced endovascular techniques. One of the advantages of robotic-assisted device control is the stable and reliable manipulation compared to manual manipulation.

The first studies regarding tele-stenting were a milestone for robotic assisted endovascular therapies. This feature can overcome the burden of patient transportation in diseases where time window dictates patient outcome like stroke management.

The interest in remote stroke interventions is especially high as it shows an increasing trend in overall US population and recent thrombectomy interventions provided significant improvement in stroke outcomes. These procedures require experienced staff and immediate action, the treatment option is currently not available for great portion of the residents because of geographical difficulties. The use of tele-robotic systems in stroke management has the capability to offer a potential solution for disseminating acute thrombectomy care to smaller regions as well.

A key factor for remote endovascular procedure is the high-speed connection in between the local and remote site this provides better communication in the medical team and also an improved endovascular robotic-assisted navigation. Performing remote robotic-assisted operation in hospitals, does not equal improvement in postoperative patient care, to be able to maintain a well-functioning center sufficient cardiovascular and neurology intensive care units are mandatory. Therefore, the widespread of remote endovascular interventions in acute patient care is theoretical.

The future generation of endovascular robotics will include broader device compatibility like 0.035-inch wires, wider-range options for guide catheters, balloons or stents. These would support the application of robotic-assisted endovascular intervention in more time-consuming procedures like contralateral gate cannulation during EVAR, target vessel catheterization and stenting in FEVAR or crossing the aortic bifurcation with the up-and-over technique.

## 7. Conclusion

CorPath system allows to perform remote endovascular procedures, promotes precise device navigation and reduces occupational hazards for the operator. Based on currently available experience the system has high procedural success rate in peripheral vascular, neurovascular and coronary interventions.

## Conflict of interest

None.

## Author details

Marton Berczeli[1,2]*, Peter Legeza[1,2] and Alan Lumsden[1]

1 Department of Cardiovascular Surgery, Houston Methodist Hospital, Houston, TX, USA

2 Department of Vascular and Endovascular Surgery, Semmelweis University, Budapest, Hungary

*Address all correspondence to: mtberczeli@houstonmethodist.org

## References


[1] Saliba W, Reddy VY, Wazni O, Cummings JE, Burkhardt JD, Haissaguerre M, et al. Atrial fibrillation ablation using a robotic catheter remote control system: initial human experience and long-term follow-up results. J Am Coll Cardiol. 2008;51(25):2407-11.

[2] Duran C, Lumsden AB, Bismuth J. A randomized, controlled animal trial demonstrating the feasibility and safety of the Magellan endovascular robotic system. Ann Vasc Surg. 2014;28(2):470-8.

[3] Schwein A, Kramer B, Chinnadurai P, Virmani N, Walker S, O'Malley M, et al. Electromagnetic tracking of flexible robotic catheters enables "assisted navigation" and brings automation to endovascular navigation in an in vitro study. J Vasc Surg. 2018;67(4):1274-81.

[4] Granada JF, Delgado JA, Uribe MP, Fernandez A, Blanco G, Leon MB, et al. First-in-human evaluation of a novel robotic-assisted coronary angioplasty system. JACC Cardiovasc Interv. 2011; 4(4):460-5.

[5] Legeza P, Britz GW, Loh T, Lumsden A. Current utilization and future directions of robotic-assisted endovascular surgery. Expert Rev Med Devices. 2020;17(9):919-27.

[6] Bordoli SJ, Carsten CG, 3rd, Cull DL, Johnson BL, Taylor SM. Radiation safety education in vascular surgery training. J Vasc Surg. 2014;59(3):860-4.

[7] Challa K, Warren SG, Danak S, Bates MC. Redundant protective barriers: minimizing operator occupational risk. J Interv Cardiol. 2009;22(3):299-307.

[8] Rolls A, Riga C. Endovascular robotics. Ann R Coll Surg Engl. 2018;100(Suppl 7): 14-7.

[9] Madder R. TCT-539 Impact of a Novel Advanced Robotic Wiring Algorithm on Time to Wire a Coronary Artery Bifurcation in a Porcine Model. In: Lombardi W, Parikh M, Kandzari D, Grantham JA, Rao S, editors. p. B223.

[10] Al Nooryani A, Aboushokka W. Rotate-on-Retract Procedural Automation for Robotic-Assisted Percutaneous Coronary Intervention: First Clinical Experience. Case Rep Cardiol. 2018;2018:6086034.

[11] Cairns E $ 1bn corindus deal gets healthineers off the acquisition blocks. Evaluate [Internet]. 2019 Aug 8 [cited 2020 Aug 20]. Available from: https://www.evaluate.com/vantage/articles/news/deals/1bn-corindus-deal-gets-healthineers-acquisition-blocks#:~:text=Corindus's%20flagship%20system%20is%20the,which%20sells%20for%20around%20%24480%2C000.

[12] Weisz G, Metzger DC, Caputo RP, Delgado JA, Marshall JJ, Vetrovec GW, et al. Safety and feasibility of robotic percutaneous coronary intervention: PRECISE (Percutaneous Robotically-Enhanced Coronary Intervention) Study. J Am Coll Cardiol. 2013;61(15):1596-600.

[13] Mahmud E, Naghi J, Ang L, Harrison J, Behnamfar O, Pourdjabbar A, et al. Demonstration of the Safety and Feasibility of Robotically Assisted Percutaneous Coronary Intervention in Complex Coronary Lesions: Results of the CORA-PCI Study (Complex Robotically Assisted Percutaneous Coronary Intervention). JACC Cardiovasc Interv. 2017;10(13):1320-7.

[14] Ellis SG, Vandormael MG, Cowley MJ, DiSciascio G, Deligonul U, Topol EJ, et al. Coronary morphologic and clinical determinants of procedural outcome with angioplasty for multivessel coronary disease. Implications for patient selection. Multivessel Angioplasty Prognosis Study Group. Circulation. 1990;82(4):1193-202.

[15] Walters D, Reeves RR, Patel M, Naghi J, Ang L, Mahmud *E. Complex* robotic compared to manual coronary interventions: 6- and 12-month outcomes. Catheter Cardiovasc Interv. 2019;93(4):613-7.

[16] Patel TM, Shah SC, Soni YY, Radadiya RC, Patel GA, Tiwari PO, et al. Comparison of Robotic Percutaneous Coronary Intervention With Traditional Percutaneous Coronary Intervention: A Propensity Score-Matched Analysis of a Large Cohort. Circ Cardiovasc Interv. 2020;13(5):e008888.

[17] Bismuth J, Duran C, Stankovic M, Gersak B, Lumsden AB. A first-in-man study of the role of flexible robotics in overcoming navigation challenges in the iliofemoral arteries. J Vasc Surg. 2013;57(2 Suppl):14S-9S.

[18] Mahmud E, Schmid F, Kalmar P, Deutschmann H, Hafner F, Rief P, et al. Feasibility and Safety of Robotic Peripheral Vascular Interventions: Results of the RAPID Trial. JACC Cardiovasc Interv. 2016;9(19):2058-64.

[19] Mahmud E, Schmid F, Kalmar P, Deutschmann H, Hafner F, Rief P, et al. Robotic Peripheral Vascular Intervention With Drug-Coated Balloons is Feasible and Reduces Operator Radiation Exposure: Results of the Robotic-Assisted Peripheral Intervention for Peripheral Artery Disease (RAPID) Study II. J Invasive Cardiol. 2020;32(10):380-4.

[20] Behnamfar O, Pourdjabbar A, Yalvac E, Reeves R, Mahmud E. First Case of Robotic Percutaneous Vascular Intervention for Below-the-Knee Peripheral Arterial Disease. J Invasive Cardiol. 2016;28(11):E128-E31.

[21] Majewska N, Blaszak MA, Juszkat R, Frankiewicz M, Makalowski M, Majewski W. Patients' radiation doses during the implantation of stents in carotid, renal, iliac, femoral and popliteal arteries. Eur J Vasc Endovasc Surg. 2011;41(3):372-7.

[22] Caputo R, Lesser A, Simons A. CRT-313 Feasibility of Robotic Percutaneous Renal Artery Revascularization. JACC: Cardiovascular Interventions. 2015;8(2_Supplement): S35-S6.

[23] Pourdjabbar A, Ang L, Reeves RR, Patel MP, Mahmud E. The Development of Robotic Technology in Cardiac and Vascular Interventions. Rambam Maimonides Med J. 2017;8(3).

[24] Cochennec F, Kobeiter H, Gohel M, Marzelle J, Desgranges P, Allaire E, et al. Feasibility and safety of renal and visceral target vessel cannulation using robotically steerable catheters during complex endovascular aortic procedures. J Endovasc Ther. 2015;22(2):187-93.

[25] Riga CV, Bicknell CD, Hamady MS, Cheshire NJ. Evaluation of robotic endovascular catheters for arch vessel cannulation. J Vasc Surg. 2011;54(3): 799-809.

[26] Perera AH, Riga CV, Monzon L, Gibbs RG, Bicknell CD, Hamady M. Robotic Arch Catheter Placement Reduces Cerebral Embolization During Thoracic Endovascular Aortic Repair (TEVAR). Eur J Vasc Endovasc Surg. 2017;53(3):362-9.

[27] Jones B, Riga C, Bicknell C, Hamady M. Robot-Assisted Carotid Artery Stenting: A Safety and Feasibility Study. Cardiovasc Intervent Radiol. 2021.

[28] Britz GW, Panesar SS, Falb P, Tomas J, Desai V, Lumsden A. Neuroendovascular-specific engineering modifications to the CorPath GRX Robotic System. J Neurosurg. 2019:1-7.

[29] Sajja KC, Sweid A, Al Saiegh F, Chalouhi N, Avery MB, Schmidt RF, et al. Endovascular robotic: feasibility and proof of principle for diagnostic cerebral angiography and carotid artery stenting. J Neurointerv Surg. 2020;12(4):345-9.

[30] Mendes Pereira V, Cancelliere NM, Nicholson P, Radovanovic I, Drake KE, Sungur JM, et al. First-in-human, robotic-assisted neuroendovascular intervention. J Neurointerv Surg. 2020;12(4):338-40.

[31] Britz GW, Tomas J, Lumsden A. Feasibility of Robotic-Assisted Neurovascular Interventions: Initial Experience in Flow Model and Porcine Model. Neurosurgery. 2020;86(2):309-14.

[32] Tsafrir Z, Janosek-Albright K, Aoun J, Diaz-Insua M, Abd-El-Barr AE, Schiff L, et al. The impact of a wireless audio system on communication in robotic-assisted laparoscopic surgery: A prospective controlled trial. PLoS One. 2020;15(1):e0220214.

[33] Madder RD, VanOosterhout S, Parker J, Sconzert K, Li Y, Kottenstette N, et al. Robotic telestenting performance in transcontinental and regional pre-clinical models. Catheter Cardiovasc Interv. 2020.

[34] Madder RD, VanOosterhout S, Mulder A, Bush J, Martin S, Rash AJ, et al. Network latency and long-distance robotic telestenting: Exploring the potential impact of network delays on telestenting performance. Catheter Cardiovasc Interv. 2020;95(5):914-9.

[35] Madder RD, VanOosterhout S, Mulder A, Bush J, Martin S, Rash A, et al. Feasibility of robotic telestenting over long geographic distances: a pre-clinical ex vivo and in vivo study. EuroIntervention. 2019;15(6):e510-e2.

[36] Patel TM, Shah SC, Pancholy SB. Long Distance Tele-Robotic-Assisted Percutaneous Coronary Intervention: A Report of First-in-Human Experience. EClinicalMedicine. 2019;14:53-8.

Chapter 7

# Present Challenges of Robotics in Gynecology

*Pranjal H. Desai and Ryan J. Gillentine*

## Abstract

Hysterectomy is one of the most common operations performed in gynecology. In the last decade and a half, the da Vinci robotic system has gained widespread acceptance in gynecology due to enhanced visualization and excellent dexterity compared to conventional laparoscopic techniques. The rapid adoption of the technology comes with unique challenges. Excluding initial acquisition cost and maintenance cost, surgery performed robotically is expensive than laparoscopic surgery. Higher cost on each case questions many about the viability of the robotic platform. Several hospitals have successfully established the robotic program, but many are reluctant to acquire expensive technology, and some are rolling back on their decision due to various reasons. This chapter expands on those challenges, mainly needs assessment, team building, culture of safety, learning curve, business strategy, and return of investment.

**Keywords:** Robotic hysterectomy, need assessment, team building, learning curve, culture of safety, business model

## 1. Introduction

Hysterectomy is the surgical procedure to remove the uterus surgically. The word 'Hysterectomy' is invented based on Ancient Greek hustéra, "womb" and ektomía- "a cutting out of," and, thus, means the removal of the uterus. Hysterectomies can be performed by open incision, vaginally, or minimally invasively—either by laparoscopy or robotically. Around 600,000 hysterectomies are performed in the United States annually [1]. Out of them, 85% are for non-cancerous lesions [2]. The traditional open approach to perform hysterectomies involves making a large incision around 10–15 cm above the pubic bone horizontally or vertically. Studies have demonstrated that hysterectomies with open approaches have higher blood loss, increased average length of hospital stay, and more postoperative complications in comparison to minimal invasive approach, including laparoscopic and robotic. The laparoscopic approach has been used for more than three decades and has become standard of care for many gynecological procedures. In 2005, the US Food and Drug Administration approved the use of the da Vinci robotic system for gynecologic surgeries. The use of this technology has allowed surgeons to perform gynecologic procedures with improvements in visualization, including 3D stereoscopic visualization, increased range of motion with enhanced wrist movements, and improved ergonomics with excellent dexterity compared to conventional laparoscopic techniques [3, 4]. However, studies have not shown any difference in operative or postoperative outcomes for patients undergoing robotic hysterectomies compared to laparoscopic hysterectomies [5, 6]. The robotic approach, indeed, has longer operative times [7] for certain operations and is more expensive, not exclusively limited to only operative cost (6–25% more than laparoscopy) [8] but also initial acquisition cost and maintenance cost compared to the standard laparoscopic approach [9]. The da Vinci system requires an initial investment of $1.5 to $2.5 million, depending on the model and configuration. Ongoing costs include annual service contracts (ranging in price from $150 to $170 K), instrument and accessory costs (ranging from $700–$3,500 per procedure).

Despite all shortcomings, surgeons still appreciate excellent visualization providing [6] more precision in surgery and better ergonomics, allowing them to do certain complex tasks, which would be very difficult with standard laparoscopic procedure. Many studies have shown the utility of the robotic platform with better outcomes and safety profiles for various benign conditions, including robotic myomectomies [10] for fibroids, robotic-assisted laparoscopic sacrocolpopexy for pelvic organ prolapse, endometriosis, benign ovarian tumors, etc. [7, 10]. The role of minimally invasive surgery for endometrial cancer has been well established by LAP 2 study [11, 12]. In addition, the role of robotic platform for other gynecological cancer including early cervical and ovarian cancer have been investigated as well [13]. In 2012, the Clinical Practice Robotics Task Force of the Society of Gynecologic Oncology stated that robotic-assisted surgery in the field of gynecology-oncology provides an advantage over traditional methods, including conventional laparoscopic approaches and laparotomies [14]. The use of robotic platform has been well established in many gynecological procedures and in other specialties like general surgery, urology, cardiothoracic surgery, etc. However, with higher acquisition and maintenance costs and with no difference in reimbursement compared to the standard laparoscopic procedure, many small community hospitals that initially acquired a robotic platform by using all cash reserves are struggling to keep it going, and many are rolling back on their decision in 1–3 years [8, 15]. In addition to a higher financial burden, many other factors are roadblocks for widespread implementation or failures of robotic programs. In this article, we would like to expand further on these roadblocks and provide reasonable, evidence-based solutions.

## 2. Need assessment

Prior to the acquisition of highly expensive robotic technology, 'Need Assessment' is an imperative step for hospitals, especially small community hospitals with limited cash reserve. Despite the rapid rise of robotic surgery, its usefulness, mainly attributed to cost concern in gynecological surgeries, has been questioned by many [16]. However, to compete with the current market and other hospitals, regional hospitals have to enter into a 'medical arms race" to acquire a robotic platform [17]. Since more and more trainees graduating from residency programs are trained on a robotic platform, small community hospitals view da Vinci as a survival tool to retain and/or recruit surgeons which will keep them in business. It is not an uncommon belief among administrators that a robotic platform can be used as a marketing tool to attract more patients. Medicare in the US helps to absorb the partial cost of robotic systems for critical access hospitals based on the number of the patients on Medicare using those facilities. However, that partial cost may still be too much for the small community hospital with scarce resources to spend. Therefore, they should have to have a thorough 'need assessment' to determine whether the purchase of a robotic system is worth a 'buy.' 'Need Assessment' is a standard industry procedure routinely being carried out in large businesses to analyze the 'need,' which is the gap between the current condition and the desired

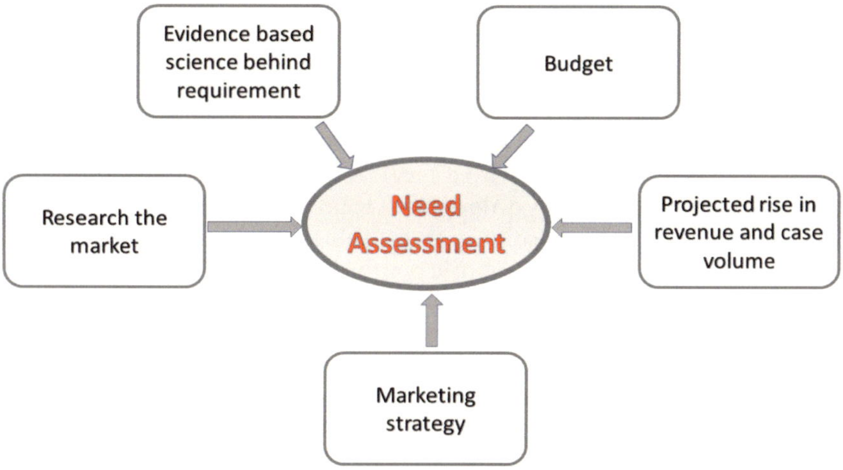
Evidence based science behind requirement
Budget
Research the market
Need Assessment
Projected rise in revenue and case volume
Marketing strategy

**Figure 1.**
*Important factors for need assessment.*

condition. Need assessment to acquire costly surgical instruments is a multistep process [18] including confirmation of necessity or define the need to acquire technology from surgeons based on evidence-based science, research the market, budget, projected rise in revenue, and room for a potential marketing strategy to increase payer mix. It is essential that hospitals should investigate the readiness of their surgeons to get trained, or hospitals should be recruiting new surgeons who are already trained. Many hospitals hire independent agencies to perform market research and viability analysis to find a sweet spot. Regardless, market research involving a rise in case volume by getting new patients who may otherwise travel far to undergo robotic procedure and internal research to determine the proportion of current surgeries which can be performed using a robotic platform are two extremely important data points in decision making. Balancing resource spending and budgeting is an integral part of the financial health of any institution, and, especially, small community hospitals walking on the thin and sharp edge of the sword. In addition to cost-effectiveness, hospitals should focus on hammering down the training program not only limited to surgeons but the entire operating room team. Finally, quite often, a hospital system which acquires the da Vinci should understand that marketing is the key to success for the program [19]. The absence of a marketing plan in place often becomes the reason for the failure of the program [20]. Therefore, research performed well in advance to investigate potential avenues of marketing strategies addressing demography or geographical needs must be well thought out prior to acquiring the system in the need assessment phase. Need Assessment phase is not only limited to investigating and analyzing the need for the da Vinci system (**Figure 1**) but also the initial planning and strategy development phase, so that when the system is acquired, administration and the entire team have a clear vision and direction of how they will be developing the program moving forward.

## 3. Team building - the cornerstone of a robotic program often neglected

Teams in the operating room have conventionally been trained in traditional open or laparoscopic surgery where the flow of the surgery is largely directed by surgeons. The mere presence of the da Vinci platform in the operating room changes many aspects of surgery as we know it, including the dynamics of the operating room along with the order of events preoperatively, intraoperatively, and postoperatively. In robotic surgery, the surgeon sits on a robotic console almost 5–10 feet away from the patient. The absence of the surgeon at the patient's bedside adds additional complexity and anxiety in the operating room among the team members. These new arrangements, including surgeon console, robotic arms, and robotic tower, require an operating room with a surgical team that is well-trained and understands the intricacies that go along with robotic surgeries, as well as the ability to share the burden of problem-solving and troubleshooting any issues that may arise throughout the process. The robotic platform brings unique challenges for the team. For instance, in nonrobotic surgery, surgeons often communicate with their team by signaling or often using not more than a single word [21]. Many a time, assistants understand the need before the surgeon even utters a word. However, in a robotic procedure, communication involves more detailed and clear instructions like pilots communicating with each other or with a control room, and everything needs to be loud and clear. The team needs to be trained to have effective bilateral communication and acknowledgment of all the instructions given by the surgeon or other way around. While traditional surgery has somewhat painted operating rooms as very strict and technical with the surgeon as the chief of events, the robotics platform enforces more of a team approach with a unique chronology of events. Thus, building an efficient team is very crucial for the success of a robotic program. This aspect can often be overlooked by either the hospital administration, the surgeon, or the operating room team. This may be overlooked because the territory of minimally invasive surgery seems familiar, but there remains the aspect of the robotic platform, which is not so familiar including the change in dynamics of the operating room with the integration of robotics. Therefore, the ability to have a successful robotic program depends not only on a surgeon who is well-versed in these technologies and surgical processes, but also a team made of members who feel like they too are an integral part of the robotic program.

Adoption of properly designed curriculum-based training is extremely important. This training should be subjected to all team members, including console surgeon, anesthesiologist, bedside assistance, assistance holding the uterine manipulator, and circulator. Initial training should include set up, docking, undocking, emergency shut down, and both mechanical and electrical troubleshooting [22]. Further training should be procedure-specific, and surgeons need to be involved in training the staff [23]. Some challenges come into play when trying to effectively build a team capable of performing these robotic procedures correctly and efficiently. For one, the surgeon must play the role of both the leader of the surgical procedure along with the leader who can effectively troubleshoot any problems which may arise through the process and can optimize operating with advanced technology. Moreover, the surgical team, including the surgeon and team members, must be willing to embrace this new technology and new approach to surgery after many years of training and practicing in ways that are totally different. A study published in Harvard Business Review by Edmonson compared 16 institutions that employed a minimally invasive approach to cardiac surgery. This study showed that some of these institutions were better able to use their experience for their advantage than others. The study demonstrated that motivation to learn was the most consistent characteristic with the ability to build a successful team, not the conventional predictors like case volume or experience level [24]. Personality traits of members of a successful team are not limited to openness to change, willingness to seek and elicit feedback, and readiness to recognize when they make a mistake. On the contrary, less successful programs employed leaders who were not as open to change and were not as effective at creating an environment conducive to learning. While this study primarily focused on cardiac surgery, the same parameters should apply to gynecologic procedures [25]. Thus, this idea of team building serves as an important cornerstone in the advancement of robotic procedures in the field of gynecologic surgery.

## 4. Culture of safety

The Institute of Medicine identifies patient safety as one of the key issues that are critical for health care delivery [26]. Changes to practice patterns that are well-established and proven to be effective always raise concerns about how they affect the safety of the patient. The same is true, to maybe an even higher degree, in the process of implementing complex and advanced technologies like robotic-assisted surgical procedures. These concerns come from healthcare personnel in every aspect of the patients' care, including operating room staff, perioperative nursing staff, anesthesia team members, and many others. While these concerns may be unfounded and unproven, they could affect morale and consequently patient outcomes [27]. Often, many hospitals implement Enhanced Recovery After Surgery (ERAS) program with robotic procedures. Many surgeons discharge robotic hysterectomy in a few hours after surgery. Nursing staff who are traditionally trained to keep minimal invasive surgery patients at least one-night inpatient may feel a little less safe to operate Enhanced Recovery After Surgery (ERAS) program and help to discharge patients home in few hours after major surgery. Studies have found that teamwork and collaboration, meetings to provide opportunities for clarification [28, 29], and staff education [30, 31] are key elements for the success of ERAS, which again supports our argument to develop an adequate culture of safety by proper communications with all stakeholders involved in postoperative care, including patients. Similarly, this has been shown in several studies that have shown that scoring higher on questions about teamwork and better communication/co-ordination is correlated with shorter length of stay and associated postoperative morbidities and mortalities. A study by Hughes et al. highlighted that 40% of US hospital nursing staff think that making changes to make improvements is difficult most of the time or all the time, which is very relevant to the implementation of advanced technologies in medical practice [32]. Recognizing that errors are sometimes inevitable, incorporating nonpunitive error reporting and analysis systems, a platform for open discussion, a willingness to learn from errors, and identifying latent threats are all characteristics of strong cultures of safety.

Three vital organizational factors are responsible for a strong environment of culture of safety: (1) environmental structures and processes within the organization, (2) the attitudes and perceptions of workers, and (3) the safety-related behaviors of individuals [33]. Institute of Medicine (US) Committee on the Work Environment for Nurses and Patient Safety narrated the following essential elements of an effective safety culture. These include a commitment of leadership to safety, empowerment and engagement of all employees in ongoing vigilance, communication, non-hierarchical decision making, constrained improvisation, training, confidential error reporting, fair and just responses to reported errors, reporting near misses as well as errors, etc. [34]. Two major barriers have been identified in adopting culture of safety. First is 'A nursing culture that fosters unrealistic expectations of clinical perfection.' Nurses are trained to believe that there is no alternative to clinical perfection, and error is the result of their carelessness that makes them less than good nurses. Higher standards and error-free care are always appreciated, but when that belief becomes counterproductive, it affects the overall care and goals of any program. Therefore, it is imperative to communicate with nurses that error is a systemic problem and not an individual one. Their minds need to be trained not to think any less of their colleagues when they make errors. Second is 'litigation and regulatory barriers.' Unfortunately, regulatory boards and the court of law or peer review processes at hospitals again reinforce the idea of clinical perfection. Therefore, it is very difficult for nursing staff to deviate from the routine practice and adopt changes that come with new technology. The culture of safety will play a large role in the outcomes of robotic-assisted surgeries, and therefore, it is both necessary and vital to address the changes that come with the implementation of novel technology. To develop a successful robotic program, it is important to implement frequent reviews of outcomes, multidisciplinary discussions, development of parameter-based new postoperative care protocols, and consideration of recommendations and management strategies from all the team members. This is a crucial part of the process of building a gynecologic surgical robotic program, and it requires commitment from members at all levels in the health care delivery system with a strong sense of culture of safety.

## 5. Learning curve

In 1885, German psychologist Herman Ebbinghaus described the concept of the learning curve, saying, "By a sufficient number of repetitions their final mastery is ensured [35]". In 1936, Wright endorsed the concept of the learning curve by hypothesizing that by increasing production one achieves perfection and, consequently, requires less time to produce aircrafts. Over 1,200 robotic programs have been established across the United States, with over 1,500 gynecologic surgeons being trained in the technology. Along with this training, there obviously comes a learning curve. This phenomenon is well-established with robotic surgery in all specialties, and multiple studies have been published to discuss the learning curve and minimum cases require to surpass the learning curve [36, 37]. The learning curve could be different for surgeons with advanced surgical skills [38] and variable for different portions of the same surgical procedure [39]. Acquisition and maintenance of a robotic program is a costly venture [16]. Not including initial acquisition, robotic hysterectomies cost roughly $2000 more than laparoscopic hysterectomies. This increased cost difference is attributed to the cost of instruments (Intuitive surgical has restricted the number of instruments in use), the costs of operating room time, costs of staffing, costs of training, and costs of personal egos. Out of these, the learning curve certainly accounts for the costs of increased operating room time, costs of personal egos, costs of the number of instruments used, costs associated with complications, etc. Therefore, before adopting a robotic program, surgeons and hospital administration should have proper understanding of the phenomenon of 'the learning curve," and its implications on the balance sheet of the hospitals. Typically, the learning curve has been described as an S-curve or sigmoid shape (**Figure 2A**). The Y-axis represents learning, and the x-axis represents experience. Classical sigmoid behavior represents an initially slow, then rapid, and subsequently slow improvement [40]. In most medical studies of learning curves, the statistical approach discretizes cases into groups and uses standard statistical methods to compare the variables. This methodology provides the statistical significance values, but it is not always the optimal way to assess the learning curve which is a dynamic process in which improvement occurs on a case-to-case basis.

A sensitive way to portray surgical failures that are indicative of both the early learning curve and the post-learning curve is the cumulative sum failure analysis (CUSUM) [41–43]. This technique not only recognizes time as an important, hidden

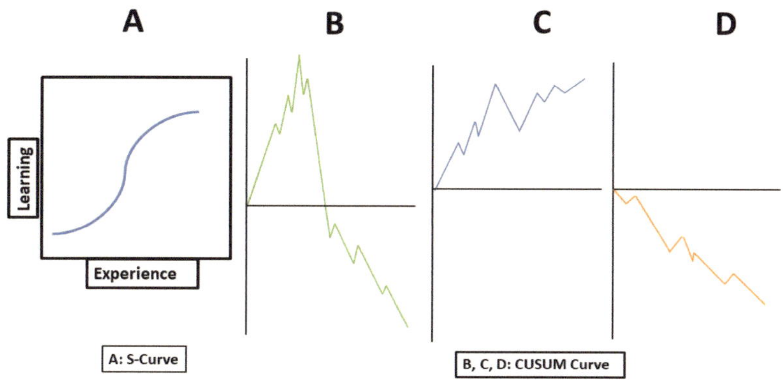


**Figure 2.**
*Learning curve. A - S curve; B, C, D - different type of hypothetical CUSUM curve.*

variable in these studies, but it also prevents the decreased statistical significance that can sometimes accompany repeat testing. For these reasons, both the standard statistical method and cumulative sum analysis are recommended to fully assess new teams with accurate and objective feedback. The following formula is used to plot the cumulative sum curve: Sn = Σ(Xi–Xo) where Xi = 0 means success and Xi = 1 means failure. Xo represents the predicted risk of major adverse events. The X-axis portrays the number of cases, while the Y-axis represents the sum of failure. This is shown in the figure (**Figure 2B**). The line that trends above the baseline portrays the learning curve or a performance that does not meet expectations. Contrarily, the line trending toward or below the baseline portrays the performance that is improving or the post-learning curve, respectively. The line trending below the baseline and away from the baseline shows adequate experience or performance that is either better or equivocal. Examples of these graphs are represented in **Figures 2B–D**. **Figure 2A** shows the analysis of a hypothetical CUSUM analysis of any successful procedure as explained above. **Figure 2C** has a curve above and moving away from the baseline. This could represent an example of either an unsuccessful procedure or a surgeon not passing the learning curve. **Figure 2D** shows the curve representing either a surgeon with excellent skills from the beginning or having escaped the learning curve that happens when skillful laparoscopic surgeons start performing robotic cases. The assessment of learning not only plays a critical role in development of an effective robotics program to assess the initial learning curve, but it also provides continued monitoring by assessing the state of the learning curve of the entire division from time-to-time which is a critical part of a robotic program [44].

## 6. Business perspective and return on investment (ROI)

The most important step in acquiring technology is the financial willingness of administration to invest in advanced technology. Therefore, understanding the business model associated with a robotic program is critical. Unlike other industries, the healthcare industry has not experienced a paradigm shift from long-term strategies to transient gain primarily due to the lengthy process that new medical and surgical advancements must undergo to be accepted as a new standard of care. To keep steady profits, companies employ many strategies. One of the strategies is to reduce costs by increasing production and providing the most cost-effective products to market. They often use the theory of "planned obsolescence" [45] by making products with reduced artificial lifespan and, thereby, get repeat sales. One of the most effective strategies is eliminating the competition, so companies can dictate the prices to their buyers. At present, Intuitive Inc. is the only company that produces viable robotic technology approved for human use and unilaterally decides the production cost, maintenance cost, cost of equipment and other accessories, etc. Therefore, administrators have only limited room to save money by reducing operating time, turn-over time, and the costs associated with readmissions and complications. On average, 150 to 300 cases annually are required for at least six years to offset the initial and ongoing costs of the da Vinci System [46]. **Figure 3** shows five industry-tested steps are important to understand in implementation of a robotic program from a business standpoint. It is also important for administrators to understand that competitive advantage is not sustainable, and therefore, requires an evolution in business strategies over time. Thus, it is important to both monitor and incentivize the upscaling phase along with maximizing both the exploitation and reconfiguration stages to further optimize return on investment (ROI) in advanced surgical technology.

Recently, a study analyzed 180,230 women who underwent laparoscopic or robotic-assisted laparoscopic hysterectomies for either benign or malignant indications (specifically endometrial cancer) from 2006 to 2012 [47]. This study demonstrated that the cost of robotic-assisted hysterectomy remained high, but this cost is offset by increased procedure volume. The use of robotic assisted technology was also found to decrease cost for oncology cases but not in benign gynecological surgeries. The cost difference between hysterectomies performed by three different modalities was analyzed by Bell and colleagues [48]. Data reveals that on average, compared to robotic procedures, the total cost for hysterectomies with staging was approximately 30–40% higher in the procedures completed by laparotomy ($P < .005$), but robotic was 10% more expensive than laparoscopic surgeries ($P = NS$). It can be hypothesized that during the phase of the learning curve, there would be major cost burdens associated with the time of the operation, turn over time, initial complications, prolonged hospital stays for some cases, conversions to open laparotomy, and overhead costs associated with the initial cost of acquisition.

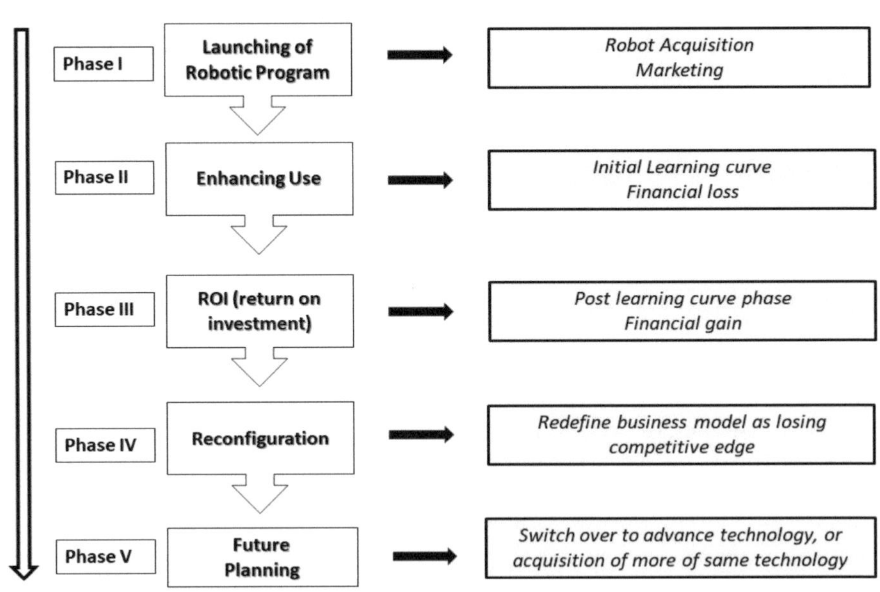


**Figure 3.**
*Five important steps in implementation of a robotic program from business standpoint.*

Due to these increased cost burdens, this would potentially minimize the cost advantage of robotic-assisted surgeries over the traditional laparotomy throughout the learning period.

After studying various case studies and industry best practices, we proposed a three-stage business model for a robotic program: 1) Negative earning, 2) Zero sum, and 3) Positive earnings (**Figure 4**). The stage of negative earnings coincides with the initial learning curve stage. Hospital administrators should have strategies in place to overcome the expected financial losses during this time. The most important strategies include low-risk case selections (which would typically offer better outcomes and minimize risks of potential losses) and thereby ensuring excellent patient satisfaction (which would lead to popularity and recognition of the program and strengthen the morale of the surgical staff) and continuous monitoring of the learning curve by various parameters such as operating time (used by surgeons), pre-docking and post-docking time (typically used by nursing and anesthesia), turn over time (time required from the end of one case to the beginning of next case), complications, length of stay, etc. In the zero sum stage, transitioning from the learning stage to the experience stage, it should be vital to market the program with positive patient outcomes. Studies have shown [49] that more than 80% of internet users perform research to use information to make decisions regarding their health care choices, especially surgeries. After the learning curve has been conquered and the program is in the stage of positive earning, administrators can expect to acquire advantages such as expanding the payer mix, which will include more private payers in addition to Medicare and Medicaid. Robotic surgery is associated with an early return to work. Private employers may be more likely to appreciate an employee's early return to work after a surgical procedure. That may provide leverage to hospitals to negotiate contracts that can bring to higher reimbursement for those procedures. Periodically, a review of outcomes and protocols associated with credentialing and recredentialing should always be performed by a multidisciplinary team to maintain safety standards and to avoid 'negligent credentialing claims' which has been increasing in the last decades in the court of law [50]. In current, profit-driven health care economics, disciplined planning, efficient strategy, and forecasting business models are the foundation for successful robotic program.

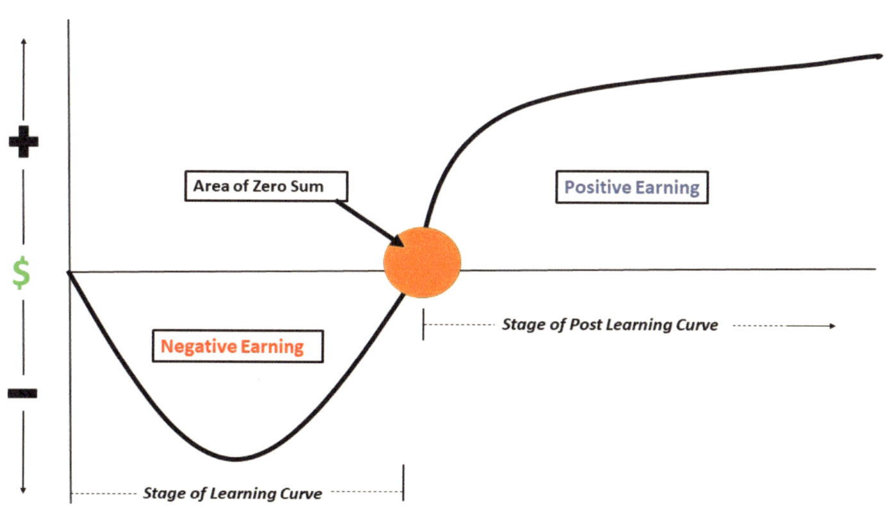


**Figure 4.**
*Hypothetical business model demonstrating sensitivity of revenue stream to learning curve.*

## 7. Conclusion

In conclusion, the adoption of a widespread robotics program for gynecological surgeries has barriers to overcome. The proposed article outlines those barriers and solutions based on literature review and our own experience. It is imperative for hospital administrators and surgeons to understand those barriers to avoid premature frustrations and proper planning for a successful robotic program to avoid the risk of suboptimal patient care and closure of the program before even it starts generating the revenue. With current health care economics, return on investment is an important concept when funds are limited, and, unlike large hospital systems with deep pockets, administrators and surgeons of small community hospital needs to understand above facts and take baby steps accordingly. Robotic platform in gynecology has continued to emerge as a very legitimate challenger to both traditional laparotomy and simple laparoscopic procedures by providing improved ergonomics and maneuvering capabilities. By overcoming the barriers outlined above, there is hope that robotic-assisted procedures will provide another legitimate option to improve outcomes for patients in the future of gynecologic operations.

## Author details

Pranjal H. Desai[1*] and Ryan J. Gillentine[2]

1 Department of Obstetrics and Gynecology, North Mississippi Medical Clinics, West Point, MS, USA

2 William Carey University College of Osteopathic Medicine, Hattiesburg, MS, USA

*Address all correspondence to: pranjaldesaiobgy@gmail.com

## References

[1] Whiteman MK, Hillis SD, Jamieson DJ, Morrow B, Podgornik MN, Brett KM, MarchbanksPA. Inpatient hysterectomy surveillance in the United States, 2000-2004. Am J Obstet Gynecol. 2008;198(1):34.e1-7. DOI: 10.1016/j.ajog.2007.05.039.

[2] Cohen SL, Vitonis AF, Einarsson JI. Updated hysterectomy surveillance and factors associated with minimally invasive hysterectomy. JSLS. 2014;18(3):e2014.00096. DOI: 10.4293/JSLS.2014.00096.

[3] Liu H, Lu D, Wang L, Shi G, Song H, Clarke J. Robotic surgery for benign gynaecological disease. Cochrane Database Syst Rev. 2012 Feb 15;(2):CD008978. DOI: 10.1002/14651858.CD008978.pub2.

[4] Maeso S, Reza M, Mayol JA, Blasco JA, Guerra M, Andradas E, Plana MN. Efficacy of the Da Vinci surgical system in abdominal surgery compared with that of laparoscopy: a systematic review and meta-analysis. Ann Surg. 2010;252(2):254-262. DOI: 10.1097/SLA.0b013e3181e6239e.

[5] Payne TN, Dauterive FR. A comparison of total laparoscopic hysterectomy to robotically assisted hysterectomy: surgical outcomes in a community practice. J Minim Invasive Gynecol. 2008;15:286-291. DOI: 10.1016/j.jmig.2008.01.008

[6] Sarlos D, Kots L, Stevanovic N, Schaer G. Robotic hysterectomy versus conventional laparoscopic hysterectomy: outcome and cost analyses of a matched case-control study. Eur J Obstet Gynecol Reprod Biol. 2010;150(1):92-96. DOI: 10.1016/j.ejogrb.2010.02.012.

[7] T Tan-Kim J, Menefee SA, Luber KM, Nager CW, Lukacz ES. Robotic-assisted and laparoscopic sacrocolpopexy: comparing operative times, costs and outcomes. Female Pelvic Med Reconstr Surg. 2011;17(1):44-49. DOI:10.1097/SPV.0b013e3181fa44cf

[8] Wright JD, Ananth CV, Lewin SN, Burke WM, Lu YS, Neugut AI, Herzog TJ, Hershman DL. Robotically assisted vs laparoscopic hysterectomy among women with benign gynecologic disease. JAMA. 2013;309(7):689-698. DOI: 10.1001/jama.2013.186.

[9] Childers CP, Maggard-Gibbons M. Estimation of the Acquisition and Operating Costs for Robotic Surgery. JAMA. 2018;320(8):835-836. DOI:10.1001/jama.2018.9219

[10] Advincula AP, Xu X, Goudeau St, Ransom SB. Robot-assisted laparoscopic myomectomy versus abdominal myomectomy: a comparison of short-term surgical outcomes and immediate costs. J Minim Invasive Gynecol. 2007;14:698-705. DOI: 10.1016/j.jmig.2007.06.008.

[11] Walker JL, Piedmonte MR, Spirtos NM, Eisenkop SM, Schlaerth JB, Mannel RS, et al. Recurrence and survival after random assignment to laparoscopy versus laparotomy for comprehensive surgical staging of uterine cancer. Gynecologic Oncology Group LAP2 Study. J Clin Oncol. 2012;30:695-700. DOI: 10.1200/JCO.2011.38.8645.

[12] Walker JL, Piedmonte MR, Spirtos NM, Eisenkop SM, Schlaerth JB, Mannel RS, et al. Laparoscopy compared with laparotomy for comprehensive surgical staging of uterine cancer. Gynecologic Oncology Group Study LAP2. J Clin Oncol. 2009;27:5331-5336. DOI: 10.1200/JCO.2009.22.3248

[13] Reynolds RK, Burke WM, Advincula AP. Preliminary experience

with robot-assisted laparoscopic staging of gynecologic malignancies. JSLS. 2005;9:149-158.

[14] Ramirez PT, Adams S, Boggess JF, Burke WM, Frumovitz MM, Gardner GJ, et al. Robotic-assisted surgery in gynecologic oncology: a Society of Gynecologic Oncology consensus statement. Developed by the Society of Gynecologic Oncology's Clinical Practice Robotics Task Force. Gynecol Oncol. 2012;124:180-184. DOI: 10.1016/j.ygyno.2011.11.006.

[15] Perez, Rafael E and S. Schwaitzberg. Robotic surgery: finding value in 2019 and beyond. Annals of Laparoscopic and Endoscopic Surgery. 2019;4:51. DOI:10.21037/ALES.2019.05.02.

[16] ACOG chairman statement---not sure how to cite this

[17] Wright JD, Tergas AI, Hou JY, Burke WM, Chen L, Hu JC, Neugut AI, Ananth CV, Hershman DL. Effect of regional hospital competition and hospital financial status on the use of robotic-assisted surgery. JAMA Surg. 2016;151(7):612-620. DOI: 10.1001/jamasurg.2015.5508.

[18] Chiappelli J. 5 steps for purchasing surgical instruments [Internet]. 2018. Available from: http://research.sklarcorp.com/5-steps-for-purchasing-surgical-instruments [Accessed 2021-02-09]

[19] Greenberg H. Marketing is key to surgical robot's success [Internet]. 2013. Available from: https://www.cnbc.com/id/100652922 [Accessed 2021-02-15]

[20] Zimmerman B. To robot or not to robot—how community hospitals can get the best robot-assisted surgery without breaking the bank [Internet]. 2018. Available from: https://www.beckershospitalreview.com/quality/to-robot-or-not-to-robot-how-community-hospitals-can-get-the-best-robot-assisted-surgery-without-breaking-the-bank.html [Accessed 2021-02-09]

[21] Lefkowitz M. Study explores how robots in the operating room impact teamwork [Internet]. 2018. Available from: https://news.cornell.edu/stories/2018/11/study-explores-how-robots-operating-room-impact-teamwork [Accessed 2021-02-09]

[22] Nifong LW, Chitwood WR, Jr. Building a surgical robotics program. The American Journal of Surgery. 2004;188(4):16-18. DOI: https://doi.org/10.1016/j.amjsurg.2004.08.026

[23] Chitwood WR Jr, Nifong LW, Chapman WH, et al. Robotic surgical training in an academic institution. Ann Surg. 2001;234(4):475-486. DOI:10.1097/00000658-200110000-00007

[24] Edmondson A, Bohmer R, Pisano G. Speeding up team learning. Harvard Bus Rev 2001;79:125-132.

[25] Desai PH, Tran R, Steinwagner T, Poston RS. Challenges of telerobotics in coronary bypass surgery. Expert Rev Med Devices. 2010;7:165-168. DOI: 10.1586/erd.09.69

[26] Kohn LT, Corrigan J, Donaldson MS. To err is human: building a safer health system. Washington (DC): National Academy Press; 2000. DOI: 10.17226/9728

[27] Singer S, Lin S, Falwell A, Gaba D, Baker L. Relationship of safety climate and safety performance in hospitals. Health Serv Res. 2009;44:399-421. DOI: 10.1111/j.1475-6773.2008.00918.x

[28] Kahokehr A, Sammour T, Zargar-Shoshtari K, Thompson L, Hill AG. Implementation of ERAS and how to overcome the barriers. Int J Surg. 2009;7(1):16-19. DOI: 10.1016/j.ijsu.2008.11.004.

[29] Gotlib Conn L, McKenzie M, Pearsall EA, McLeod RS. Successful implementation of an enhanced recovery after surgery programme for elective colorectal surgery: a process evaluation of champions' experiences. Implement Sci. 2015;10:99. DOI: 10.1186/s13012-015-0289-y.

[30] Pearsall EA, Meghji Z, Pitzul KB, Aarts MA, McKenzie M, McLeod RS, Okrainec A. A qualitative study to understand the barriers and enablers in implementing an enhanced recovery after surgery program. Ann Surg. 2015;261(1):92-96. DOI: 10.1097/SLA.0000000000000604

[31] Alawadi ZM, Leal I, Phatak UR, Flores-Gonzalez JR, Holihan JL, Karanjawala BE, Millas SG, Kao LS. Facilitators and barriers of implementing enhanced recovery in colorectal surgery at a safety net hospital: A provider and patient perspective. Surgery. 2016;159(3):700-712. DOI: 10.1016/j.surg.2015.08.025

[32] Hughes CM, Lapane KL. Nurses' and nursing assistants' perceptions of patient safety culture in nursing homes. Int J Qual Health Care. 2006;18(4):281-286. DOI: 10.1093/intqhc/mzl020

[33] Cooper M. Towards a model of safety culture. Safety Science. 2000;36:111-136.

[34] Page A, editor. Institute of Medicine (US) Committee on the Work Environment for Nurses and Patient Safety. Keeping patients safe: Transforming the work environment of nurses. Washington (DC): National Academies Press (US); 2004.

[35] Ebbinghaus H. Memory: a contribution to experimental psychology. Ann Neurosci. 2013;20(4):155-156. DOI: 10.5214/ans.0972.7531.200408

[36] Ahlering TE, Skarecky D, Lee D, Clayman RV. Successful transfer of open surgical skills to a laparoscopic environment using a robotic interface: initial experience with laparoscopic radical prostatectomy. J Urol. 2003;170(5):1738-1741. DOI: 10.1097/01.ju.0000092881.24608.5e

[37] Herrell SD, Smith JA Jr. Robotic-assisted laparoscopic prostatectomy: what is the learning curve? Urology. 2005;66(5 Suppl):105-107. DOI: 10.1016/j.urology.2005.06.084.

[38] Sammon J, Perry A, Beaule L, Kinkead T, Clark D, Hansen M. Robot-assisted radical prostatectomy: learning rate analysis as an objective measure of the acquisition of surgical skill. BJU Int. 2010;106(6):855-860. DOI: 10.1111/j.1464-410X.2009.09187.x

[39] Tang FH, Tsai EM. Learning curve analysis of different stages of robotic-assisted laparoscopic hysterectomy. Biomed Res Int. 2017;2017:1827913. DOI: 10.1155/2017/1827913

[40] Leibowitz N, Baum B, Enden G, Karniel A. The exponential learning equation as a function of successful trials results in sigmoid performance. Journal of Mathematical Psychology. 2010;54:338-340. DOI: 10.1016/j.jmp.2010.01.006.

[41] Maguire T, Mayne CJ, Terry T, Tincello DG. Analysis of the surgical learning curve using the cumulative sum (CUSUM) method. Neurourol Urodyn. 2013;32:964-967.

[42] Young A, Miller JP, Azarow K. Establishing learning curves for surgical residents using Cumulative Summation (CUSUM) Analysis. Curr Surg. 2005;62:330-334.

[43] Wohl H. The CUSUM plot: its utility in the analysis of clinical data. N Engl J Med. 1977;296:1044-1045

[44] Desai PH, Zipf E, Tchabo N, Tobias D, Ramieri J, Slomovitz B.

Establishing the stage of learning curve for robotic surgery: Institutional Cumulative Sum of Failure (CUSUM) analysis within Division of Gynecologic Oncology. Poster presented at: Society of Gynecology Oncology Annual Meeting; Austin, TX, March 2012.

[45] Hadhazy A. Here's the truth about the 'planned obsolescence' of tech [Internet]. 2016. Available from: https://www.bbc.com/future/article/20160612-heres-the-truth-about-the-planned-obsolescence-of-tech [Accessed on 2021-02-12]

[46] Lee J. Surgical-robot costs put small hospitals in a bind [Internet]. 2014. Available from: https://www.modernhealthcare.com/article/20140419/MAGAZINE/304199985/surgical-robot-costs-put-small-hospitals-in-a-bind [Accessed 2021-02-09]

[47] Wright, JD, et al. An economic analysis of robotically assisted hysterectomy. Obstet Gynecol. 2014;123(5):1038-1048.

[48] Bell MC, Torgerson J, Seshadri-Kreaden U, Suttle AW, Hunt S. Comparison of outcomes and cost for endometrial cancer staging via traditional laparotomy, standard laparoscopy and robotic techniques. Gynecol Oncol. 2008;111:407-411.

[49] Princeton Survey Research Associates International. Fall tracking survey 2008 [Internet]. 2009. Available from: https://www.pewresearch.org/internet/wp-content/uploads/sites/9/media/Files/Questionnaire/2010/PIP_Chronic_Disease-Dec08_topline.pdf [Accessed on 2021-02-12]

[50] Carreyrou J. Botched operation using da Vinci robot spurs lawsuit [Internet]. 2010. Available from: http://online.wsj.com/article/SB10001424052748703341904575266952674277806.html [Accessed on 2021-02-15]

Chapter 8

# Robotic Myomectomy: Until Achieving Reproductive Success, Step by Step

*Radamés Rivas López*

## Abstract

Surgeons who practice robotic surgery in benign gynecological conditions agree that in some cases, blood loss and transfusions are reduced, the time of hospital stay and of reintegration to daily activities is less, although commonly in the first cases of each surgeon surgical time may be longer than laparoscopic surgery depending on the learning curve of each. As in any other surgical technique, it is important that the surgeon is trained and certified in accordance with the guidelines that each hospital institution indicates for the practice of robotic surgery and is constantly updated through the tools provided by robotic surgery to ensure the correct use of this technology and always maintain the skill looking for the safety of the patient at all times. Uterine fibroids, are the most common benign tumors that appear in women of reproductive age. Depending on their location, number and size, the symptoms they produce vary in frequency and severity. Robotic myomectomy has shown that with a surgical team that operates frequently, it is superior to conventional laparoscopic myomectomy, even in the area of cost/benefit. Robotic myomectomy is an accessible, efficient and flattering pathway for patients with fibroids who want a pregnancy.

**Keywords:** leiomyoma, robotic surgery, myomectomy, infertility, myoma, fibroids, fertility

## 1. Introduction

Minimally invasive surgery is at the forefront of technology and robotic surgery is part of this new development.

This review includes the main gynecological surgeries that greatly benefit from the use of this robotic technology, such as: hysterectomy, myomectomy, tubal recanalization, sacrocolpopexy, endometriosis, and transabdominal cerclage.

Likewise, the advantages and disadvantages of this technology are analyzed, as well as the influence of the type of training and learning curve for this type of surgical approach.

Laparoscopic surgery has evolved rapidly in various specialties, in the area of gynecology, robot-assisted surgery is used in different procedures, mainly in hysterectomy for benign diseases and myomectomy, also in cases of tubal recanalization, lymphadenectomy, endometriosis and sacrocolpopexy.

Robot-assisted surgery managed to develop technical advances that surpass laparoscopic surgery such as:



IntechOpen

Vision in third dimension (3D)
High visual definition on the console
Movements of the forceps similar to those of the doctor's hand
Better ergonomic position during surgery that avoids fatigue.

Surgeons who practice robotic surgery in benign gynecological conditions agree that in some cases, blood loss and transfusions are reduced, the time of hospital stay and of reintegration to daily activities is less, although commonly in the first cases of each surgeon surgical time may be longer than laparoscopic surgery depending on the learning curve of each.

There are different opinions regarding the advantages and disadvantages that robotic surgery offers vs. laparoscopic surgery in benign gynecological conditions, which is why the advantages of this system and/or surgical approach should be known as in any other type of surgery, as well as the potential risks inherent in all surgery and notify the patient through an informed consent before the intervention.

As in any other surgical technique, it is important that the surgeon is trained and certified in accordance with the guidelines that each hospital institution indicates for the practice of robotic surgery and is constantly updated through the tools provided by robotic surgery to ensure the correct use of this technology and always maintain the skill looking for the safety of the patient at all times.

## 2. Fundamental principles to consider

Uterine fibroids, also known as fibroids or leiomyomas, are the most common benign tumors that appear in women of reproductive age. Depending on their location, number and size, the symptoms they produce vary in frequency and severity. There is scientific evidence that fibroids interfere with sperm migration, oocyte transport and embryo implantation due to endometrial inflammation or vascular alterations that they produce. Approximately 5 to 10% of infertile women have fibroids and their presence is the only abnormal factor found in up to 4% of them [1]. At present, in women of reproductive age with gestational desire and presence of fibroids, myomectomy is probably the treatment of choice.

Technology continues to evolve and expand conservative treatment options for women who desire fertility preservation. There are some techniques for this, such as: uterine artery embolization, high-frequency ultrasound guided by magnetic resonance imaging, and radiofrequency ablation. However, myomectomy remains the gold standard for women with infertility who suffer from uterine myomatosis and wish to become pregnant later [2].

The relationship between fibroids and fertility continues to be debated, especially with regard to intramural fibroids. It is generally accepted that submucosal fibroids decrease fertility and that subserous fibroids have little or no influence in this regard [3]. However, according to some reports, intramural fibroids that do not affect the cavity are also associated with unfavorable reproductive outcomes. Analysis of prospective and retrospective studies shows that intramural fibroids that do not distort the cavity have a significant adverse effect on live birth rates in women undergoing in vitro fertilization [4].

The impact of intramural fibroids that do not distort the endometrial cavity has been a point of constant controversy, especially when choosing the most appropriate therapeutic strategy, and as occurred in our study, intramural fibroids were the ones that were found more frequently in patients, without However, it is important to take into account the live birth rate and not only the postoperative pregnancy rate, since fibroids can be associated with an unfavorable obstetric outcome.

A meta-analysis carried out by Sunkara and Rikhraj years later indicated that the presence of intramural fibroids that do not distort the cavity is associated with an adverse outcome in women undergoing treatment of In Vitro Fertilization (IVF), it is mentioned that the live newborn rate in patients with fibroids is 21% lower than in women without fibroids [3, 4].

Those intramural fibroids that do not affect the cavity, the size of the same is still a point of debate, it is generally taken as a cut-off point for myomectomy those intrmaural fibroids that do not affect the cavity but are greater than or equal to 4 cm [5, 6]. As occurred in our group of patients, all intramural fibroids were at least 4 or more centimeters tall. In these cases, the route of choice for the surgical approach is preferably by minimally invasive surgery.

The surgical route of choice depends on two fundamental factors: the fibroid itself, its location, its number, size and the experience of the surgical team. Submucosal fibroids are treated hysteroscopically, while intramural and subserous fibroids can be treated laparoscopically, robotically, abdominally, or vaginally. Whenever possible, the route of choice should be through minimal access surgery, since there is a solid scientific basis in which it is shown that with the robotic laparoscopic, conventional laparoscopic or vaginal approach, there is less intraoperative blood loss, a lower rate of adhesions, less postoperative morbidity, and fewer days of hospitalization than with open myomectomy [7]. It should be noted that a recent study reported a faster return of patients to their work and/or daily activities after a myomectomy for minimally invasive surgery [8].

In this same sense, robotic myomectomy has shown that with a surgical team that operates frequently, it is superior to conventional laparoscopic myomectomy, even in the area of cost/benefit [9]. And it is that if you have a team made up of anesthesiologists, surgeons, nurses and doctors who regularly perform this type of robotic approach, efficiency, economy, shorter surgical times are achieved and the results are effective and at a reasonable cost. Even as Wu mentions, more studies are needed to determine which patients would benefit greatly from a robotic approach, both in terms of patient outcomes and cost-effectiveness [10].

Takmaz et al. It compared symptom severity and health quality outcomes for women who underwent laparoscopic and robotic myomectomy. Finding that both laparoscopic and robotic myomectomy provides significant reductions in the severity of fibroid-associated symptoms and a significant improvement in quality of life 1 year after surgery. The rate of improvement was comparable for both procedures [11].

However despite the evidence that minimally invasive surgery is preferable to laparotomy, most myomectomies are still performed by laparotomy. Robotic surgery was introduced to eliminate or improve some of the difficulties associated with laparoscopic surgery. We know that a myomectomy is a surgery that requires suturing in several planes, in different directions and with different cancelations, where it was planned that the characteristics of a surgical robot that would help to carry out this work would be of great value. Robotic myomectomy has now been shown to be efficient and safe by a vast bibliography, its results are similar to laparoscopic surgery, although the robotic procedure is associated with a higher cost. The introduction of robotic surgery has expanded the indications for minimally invasive myomectomy to more complex cases that were previously performed using laparotomy. Despite everything, and as Lonnerfors points out, no randomized, prospective and controlled trials have been published that compare the different approaches to a myomectomy in order to make an analysis and from there derive the best recommendations based on the evidence [12].

There are two meta-analyzes that can be cited, the first by Lavazzo et al. The premise was to demonstrate that robot-assisted myomectomy was an equally safe and effective treatment option as laparoscopy and open surgery for uterine myomatosis. It was found that regarding the comparison between the robotic and laparoscopic technique, no significant differences were found between both types of surgery. Concluding that the minimally invasive approach has the advantage of less blood loss, less need for transfusion and shorter hospital stay. Suggesting that long-term outcomes required clarification, including pain control, fertility, and postoperative pregnancy rates, as well as possible recurrence rates [13].

Two years later, Wang et al. They carried out a new meta-analysis on our subject and concluded that compared to the laparoscopic and abdominal approaches, robotic surgery is significantly associated with: lower indices of complications, lower conversion rate of the procedure and less operative bleeding [14].

The results in functional terms after performing a myomectomy by any approach is to achieve the birth of a healthy baby. In Mexico, the first successful report on a robot-assisted myomectomy was made by our surgical team [14]. However, in this area there are not such drastic conclusions about the approach in favor of one or another technique according to the superiority of its reproductive results and the absence of randomized studies that compare the different surgical approaches in this regard. However Jayakumaran in a comparative analysis of the role of robot-assisted laparoscopy in the field of reproductive surgery the reported advantages and limitations of the use of robotics in reproductive surgeries such as myomectomy, among others. He found that robotic assistance in reproductive surgery presented decreased blood loss, less post-operative pain, a shorter hospital stay, and a faster convalescence, while reproductive outcomes were similar in the other approaches. He likewise found that robotic surgery was as safe and effective as conventional laparoscopy, representing a totally reasonable alternative to the abdominal approach. He suggesting that procedures that are technically challenging with the Conventional laparoscopy could be performed with robotic assistance due to its advantages of better visualization and Endowrist™ movements (similar to the wrist of the human hand) that allow for precise suturing. This helps to overcome the limitations of laparoscopy, especially in complicated procedures, and can shorten the learning curve of minimally invasive surgery. Thus justifying the controlled and randomized studies that compare the short and long-term results to strengthen the role of robotic surgery in the field of reproductive surgery [15].

Regarding efficiency with good results, fundamental characteristics in surgical procedures, there is the question that up to what number of fibroids would it be possible to remove by minimally invasive surgery?(16), particularly in robotic surgery. Kim et al. They demonstrated that it is feasible to perform a robotic myomectomy in patients with up to 20 fibroids, preserving efficiency and good post-operative results, being even a faster procedure than the open myomectomy with which it was compared in the study [16, 17].

## 3. Robotic myomectomy: step by step

The first step is to have a good imaging diagnosis, with magnetic resonance imaging the ideal study at this time for this as sown in **Figure 1**. This must be interpreted correctly by the surgeon, since it is the GPS to achieve success in terms of removing the number of fibroids and planning the hysterotomy.

The second step is planning regarding the configuration of robotic ports for successful intraoperative development, taking into account the following philosophy:

In robotic myomectomy, if the objective is below the umbilical scar, we can place the robotic lens at the umbilical level. But if the objective is at the umbilical level or above it, then we need an adequate working distance of between 7 and 10 cm, depending on the case to be able to develop our work well and then the lens must be at that distance level as shown in **Figure 2**.

DOI: http://dx.doi.org/10.5772/intechopen.97880

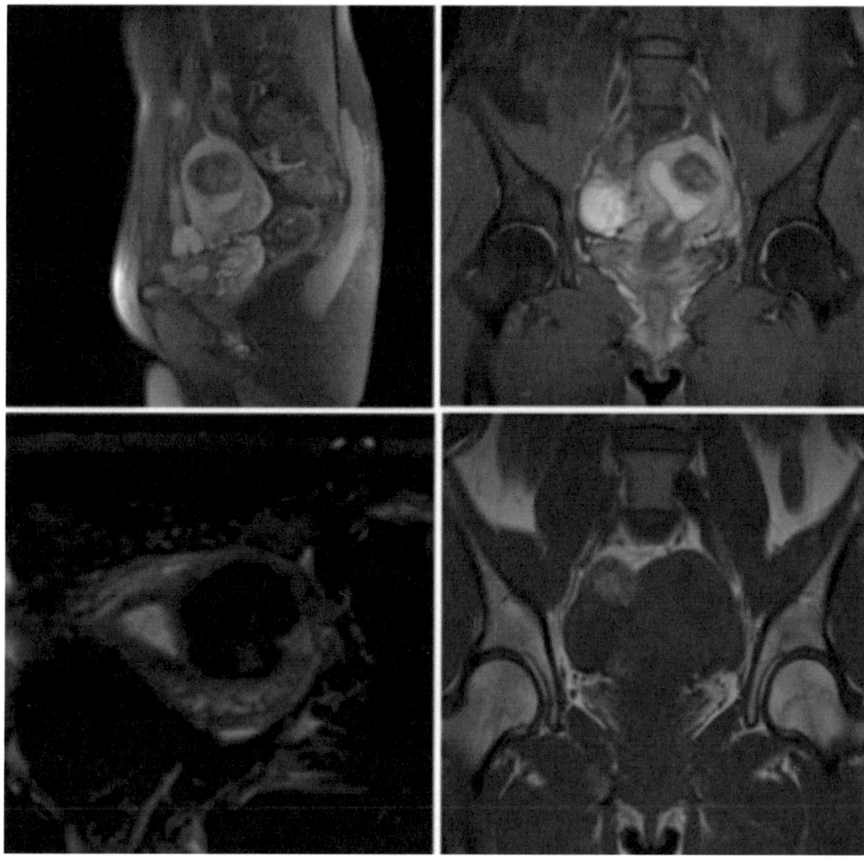

**Figure 1.**
*Protocol magnetic resonance imaging for fibroids localization.*

Finally the development of the surgery step by step is as follows:

1. Infiltration of the myometrium with dilute vasopressin. As shown in **Figure 3**.

2. Incision of the myometrium with scissors or monopolar hook in arm 1 using the monopolar energy judiciously and without excess (maximum 35 Watts). As shown in **Figure 4**.

3. Traction and countertraction technique until complete enucleation of the myoma, using a tenaculum for greater efficiency. As shown in **Figure 5**.

4. The myometrium is observed and the intact endometrial dome is observed in the center, and we do not recommend using it as much as possible as it dries and necrotic the myometrial tissue. As shown in **Figure 6**.

5. The closure of the myometrium is in three planes with preferably barbed suture that reduces operative times and reduces bleeding. As shown in **Figure 7**.

6. After the repaired uterus, hemostasis is verified. As shown in **Figure 8**.

7. At the end of the uterine suture, the robot was undocked and the fibroid was extracted by using of contained electrical or not electric morcellation. As shown in **Figure 9**.

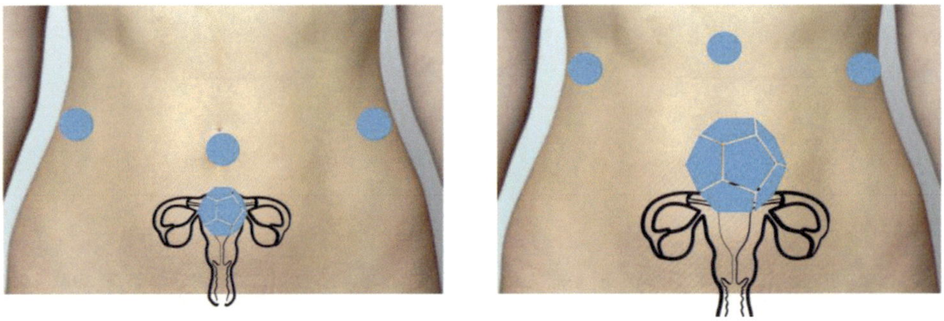

**Figure 2.**
*Port placement configuration.*

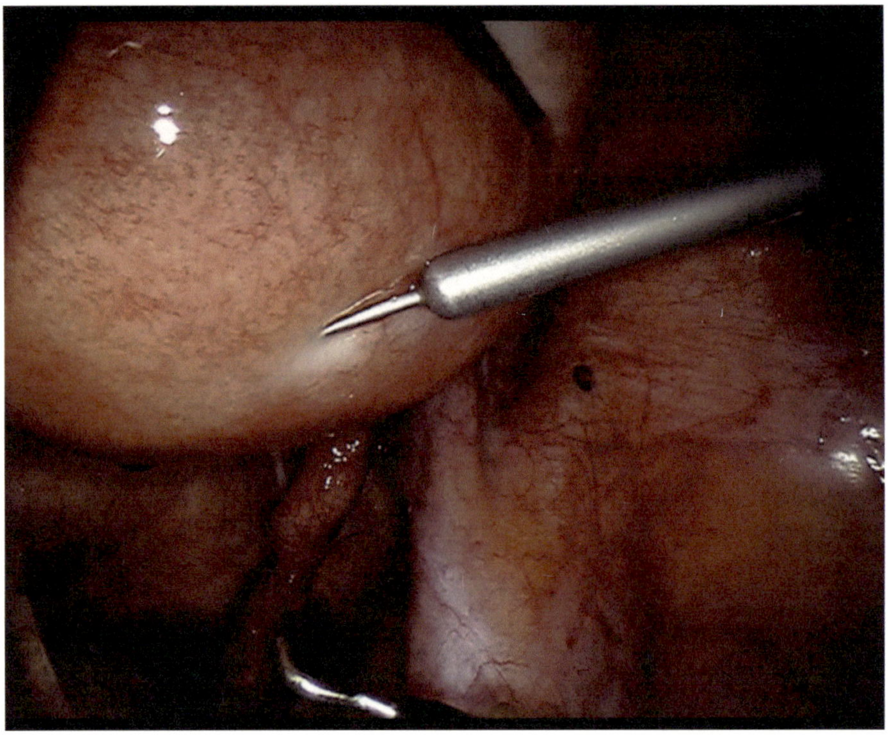

**Figure 3.**
*Infiltration of the myometrium.*

In our country there has been a good acceptance for the use of this platform in cases of myomectomies including the birth at the end of babies without the fear of a major complication such as uterine rupture. Thus showing that robotic myomectomy is an accessible, efficient and flattering pathway for patients with fibroids who want a pregnancy.

We must point out that our group performs robotic myomectomies with only two arms apart from the robot chamber, and we believe that it is essential to maintain a controlled cost in the operative processes without skimping on good results. The vast majority of the aforementioned and currently available studies have performed robotic-assisted laparoscopic myomectomies with four arms, that is, a central port for the camera and three robotic ports plus the necessary accessories, which is usually at least one. More. That gives you certain operative advantages but in most cases few cosmetic advantages and if it is to invade as little as possible

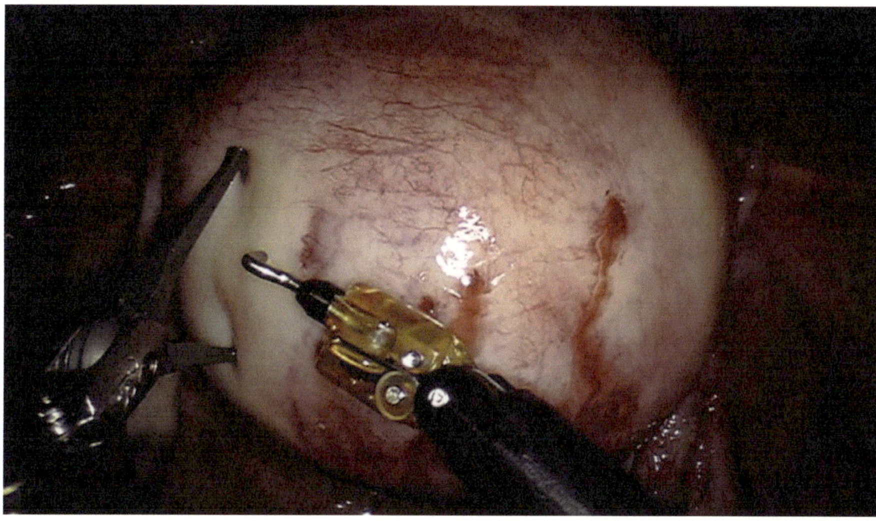

**Figure 4.**
*Incision of the myometrium.*

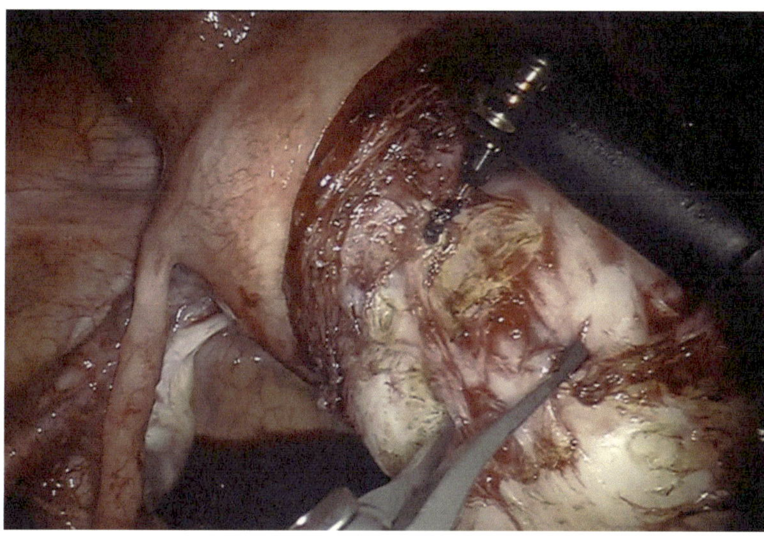

**Figure 5.**
*Myoma enucleation.*

it would be prudent to use as few ports as possible. This challenges even more any surgical plan, but provides greater esthetics, less invasion with cost containment for the benefit of all, patient, hospital and third-party payers if applicable, which is in the end what is sought, good results with minimal access.

Finally we do the following historical reflection:

1. A robot must not harm a human being or, because of its inaction, let a human being suffer harm.

2. A robot must obey orders given by a human being, except when these orders are in opposition to the first law.

3. A robot must protect its own existence, until this protection is not in conflict with the first or second laws.

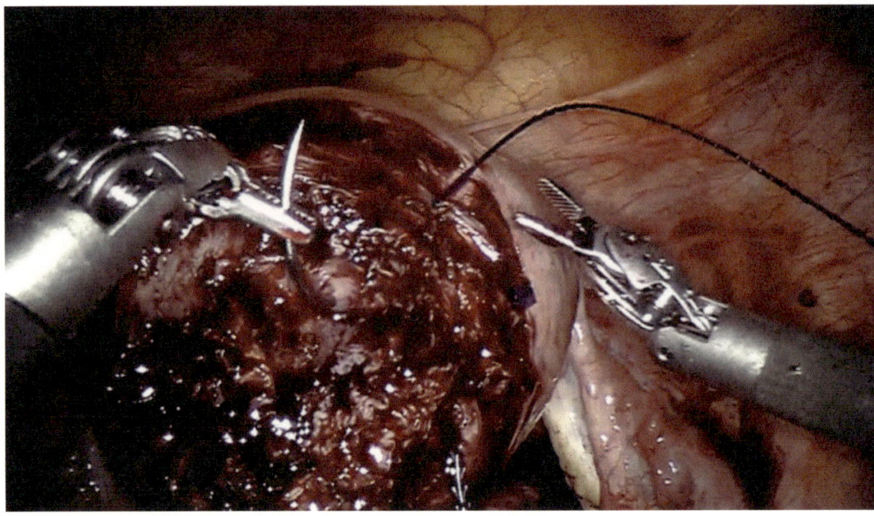

**Figure 6.**
*Intact endometrial dome and less use of energy.*

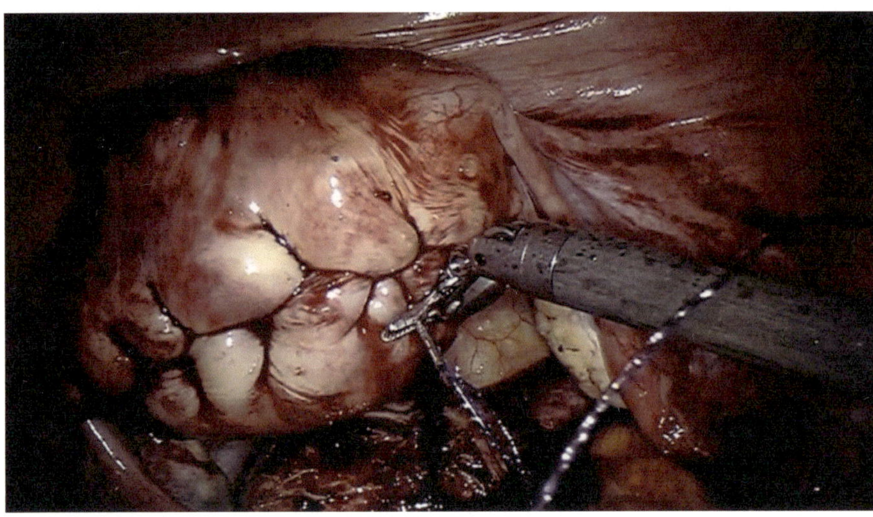

**Figure 7.**
*Total myometrium closure.*

The above is an excerpt from Isaac Asimov's futuristic novel: Me, a robot written in 1950 and showing how human beings have always maintained a special interest in the robotic theme [18]. What awaits us in the future? we will know soon.

## 4. Conclusion

Technology continues to evolve and expand conservative treatment options for women who desire fertility preservation. Whenever possible, the route of choice should be through minimal access surgery, since there is a solid scientific basis in which it is shown that with the robotic laparoscopic there is less intraoperative blood loss, a lower rate of adhesions, less postoperative morbidity, fewer days of hospitalization and a faster return of patients to their work and/or daily activities.

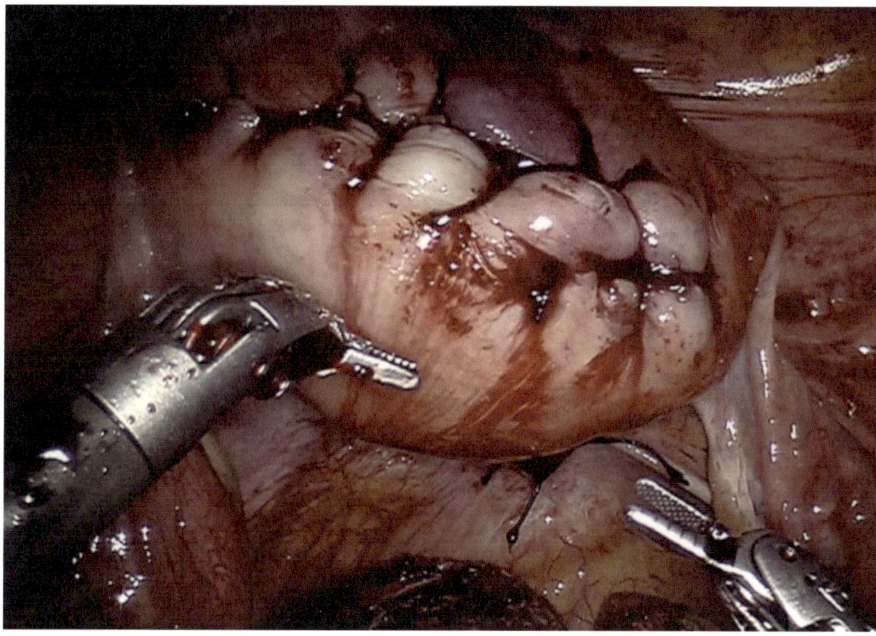

**Figure 8.**
*Verify hemostasis.*

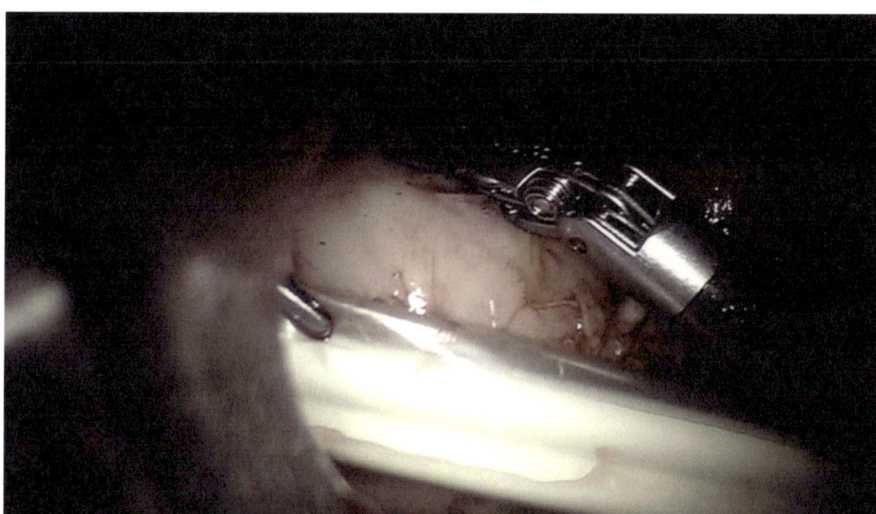

**Figure 9.**
*Contained morcelation.*

## Author details

Radamés Rivas López
The Mexican Association of Robotic Surgery and Center of Robotic Surgery, Reproductive Medicine Women's Clinic Ángeles Pedregal Hospital, México City, México

*Address all correspondence to: radamesrl@hotmail.com

## References

[1] Khaund A, Lumsden MA. Impact of fibroids on reproductive function. Best Pract Res Clin Obstet Gynaecol 2008;22(4): 749e60.

[2] Gobern JM, Rosemeyer CJ, Barter JF, Steren AJ. Comparison of robotic, laparoscopic, and abdominal myomectomy in a community hospital. *JSLS*. 2013;17(1):116-120.

[3] Cook H, Ezzati M, Segars JH, et al. The impact of uterine leiomyomas on reproductive outcomes. Minerva Ginecol 2010 Jun;62(3):225e36.

[4] Sunkara SK, Khairy M, El-Toukhy T, et al. The effect of intramural fibroids without uterine cavity involvement on the outcome of IVF treatment: a systematic review and meta-analysis. Hum Reprod 2010;25:418e29.

[5] Rikhraj K, Tan J, Taskin O, Albert AY, Yong P, Bedaiwy MA. The Impact of Noncavity-Distorting Intramural Fibroids on Live Birth Rate in *In Vitro* Fertilization Cycles: A Systematic Review and Meta-Analysis. *J Womens Health (Larchmt)*. 2020;29(2): 210-219.

[6] Pritts EA, ParkerWH, Olive DL. Fibroids and infertility: and updated systematic review of the evidence. Fertil Steril 2009; 91:1215-1223

[7] Galliano D, Bellver J, Días-García C, simón C, pedllicer A. ART and uterine pathology: how relevant is the maternal side for implantation? Hum Repd Update 2015; 21 (1):13-38

[8] Gingold JA, Gueye NA, Falcone T. Minimally Invasive Approaches to Myoma Management. *J Minim Invasive Gynecol*. 2018;25(2):237-250.

[9] Laughlin-Tommaso SK, Lu D, Thomas L, et al. Short-term quality of life after myomectomy for uterine fibroids from the COMPARE-UF Fibroid Registry. *Am J Obstet Gynecol*. 2020;222(4):345.e1-345.e22.

[10] Wu CZ, Klebanoff JS, Tyan P, Moawad GN. Review of strategies and factors to maximize cost-effectiveness of robotic hysterectomies and myomectomies in benign gynecological disease. *J Robot Surg*. 2019;13(5): 635-642.

[11] Takmaz O, Ozbasli E, Gundogan S, et al. Symptoms and Health Quality After Laparoscopic and Robotic Myomectomy. *JSLS*. 2018;22(4):e2018.00030.

[12] Lonnerfors C. Robot-assisted myomectomy. *Best Pract Res Clin Obstet Gynaecol*. 2018;46:113-119.

[13] Iavazzo C, Mamais I, Gkegkes ID. Robotic assisted vs laparoscopic and/or open myomectomy: systematic review and meta-analysis of the clinical evidence. *Arch Gynecol Obstet*. 2016;294(1):5-17.

[14] Wang T, Tang H, Xie Z, Deng S. Robotic-assisted vs. laparoscopic and abdominal myomectomy for treatment of uterine fibroids: a meta-analysis. *Minim Invasive Ther Allied Technol*. 2018;27(5):249-264.

[15] Rivas-López R, 1 Durón-Padilla R, 2 Romero-Hernández S, 3 Audifred-Salomón J, 4 Hernández-Denis JA. Miomectomía laparoscópica asistida por robot y embarazo. Reporte de caso. Ginecol Obstet Mex. 2016;84(3): 194-200

[16] Jayakumaran J, Patel SD, Gangrade BK, Narasimhulu DM, Pandian SR, Silva C. Robotic-assisted laparoscopy in reproductive surgery: a contemporary review. *J Robot Surg*. 2017;11(2):97-109.

[17] Hyunkyung Kim, et al. Robot-assisted laparoscopic myomectomy, Obstet Gynecol Sci 2018;61(1):135-141

[18] Asimov I. (1950). I, Robot. Garden City, N.Y: Doubleday.

Chapter 9

# Orthopedic Bone Drilling Robot ODRO: Basic Characteristics and Areas of Applications

*Tony Boiadjiev, George Boiadjiev, Kamen Delchev, Ivan Chavdarov and Roumen Kastelov*

## Abstract

The orthopedic manipulation "bone drilling" is the most executed one in the orthopedic surgery concerning the operative treatment of bone fractures. The drilling process is characterized by a number of input and output parameters. The most important input parameters are the feed rate [mm/s] and the drill speed [rpm]. They play significant role for the final result (the output parameters): thermal and mechanical damages of the bone tissue as well as hole quality. During the manual drilling these parameters are controlled by the surgeon on the base of his practical skills. But the optimal results of the manipulations can be assured only when the input parameters are under control during an automatic execution of the drilling process. This work presents the functional characteristics of the handheld robotized system ODRO (Orthopedic Drilling Robot) for automatic bone drilling. Some experimental results are also shown. A comparison is made between the similar systems which are known in the literature, some of which are available on the market. The application areas of ODRO in the orthopedic surgery practice are underlined.

**Keywords:** automatic bone drilling, handheld robotized surgical drill, speed control, orthopedic surgery

## 1. Introduction

The bone drilling process is a basic manipulation in the osteosynthesis of the bone fractures. Osteosynthesis is a surgical procedure, which stabilizes and joins the ends of fractured (broken) bones by mechanical devices such as metal plates, screws, pins, rods, wires. Nowadays by statistics every year about one million people in Europe need such an operation where implants into bones are inserted.

The process of bone drilling is characterized by a number of input and output parameters. The input parameters define the conditions under which the process occurs, while the output parameters determine the outcome of the process.

The input parameters as feed rate [mm/s] and drill speed [rpm] are of the greatest importance for the final result of the drilling process: thermal and mechanical damages of the bone tissue, hole quality, second cortex breakthrough detection and penetration depth in the case of bicortical bone drilling.

A large amount of researches have been published related to the influence of these parameters on the bone drilling process. Only publications, indexed in

SCOPUS, related to the bone drilling process, are above 3000 since 2000 [1], which proves the importance and relevance of researches in this area.

Most of the drilling operations in orthopedic surgery are done manually (non-automatically) by hand drills and drilling performance depends on the surgeon's manual skills and 'drilling by feeling' [2]. That means recognizing the breakthrough detection (identification of the moment of time when the drill bit exits the second cortex), working with drilling rate good enough not to cause any damages to the bone or soft tissues closed to it [3].

The influence of the subjective factor is a prerequisite for the emergence of a number of problems in manual drilling. The most significant ones are:

- Wrong recognition the breakthrough detection in bicortical bone drilling. That means risks of damage of the bone, muscles, nerves and venous tissues when the drill bit does not stop immediately after coming out of the second wall of the bone

- Thermal osteonecrosis of bone cells as a result of bone drilling process. That means reduction the implant-bone pull-out strength.

Osteonecrosis is a kind of the health status depending on various conditions which lead to bone death [4]. The result is loss of blood supply or death of bone cells. It can be classified as vascular, infective, drugs or toxins, inflammatory, congenital, autoimmune, traumatic and endocrine or metabolic. One specific kind of traumatic osteonecrosis is thermal necrosis of bone.

The question of subjective factor reduction has its answer – automatic bone drilling. The use of robots would have a significant role for eliminating or minimizing the human error.

Robot applications possibility increase in the orthopedic surgery since 2000 [5, 6] but still they are rare in usage for the sake of their high cost. For example, ROBODOC (Curexo Technology Corp.) is applied for hip joint arthroplasty and costs 600 000 $ while RIO (MAKO Surgical Corp.) - 1 000 000 $ [7]. Nevertheless, the operation costs in social aspect decrease: patient recovery period is less than conventional one; complexity of the surgeon's manipulations and the risk of his potential errors become smaller [8]. On the other hand, the robot application in surgery requires specific maintenance and training of the medical staff aiming to guarantee the patient safety.

The first efforts for robot application in the orthopedic surgery are based on the industrial manipulating systems. The advanced tendency is oriented to a design of manipulative systems according to the specifics of concrete orthopedic manipulations aiming maximally simplification of robot mechanics [9, 10].

Thus so called Handheld Robotized Systems appear [11]. The handheld robotized systems answer entirely or partially to the definitions of robot [12] and robotic surgery nowadays has accepted the definition [13] of the Society of American Gastrointestinal and Endoscopic Surgeons and Minimally Invasive Robotic Association (SAGES–MIRA) Robotic Consensus Group.

The purpose of handheld robotized systems development is to reach the accuracy and precise working of the stationary multifunctional robots. Currently the following devices are available on the market and in the orthopedic surgery practice:

- handheld robotic device **SMARTdrillR**

It is developed by US Company SMD Inc. (Smart Medical Devices) and first time is presented in 2017. It measures the hole depth in real time and eliminates the plunge after the far cortex [14, 15]. SMARTdrillR has two motors: for rotation and for linear translation of the drill bit along the drilling direction. The data transfer between the SMARTdrillR and its control system is wireless. The drill bit and bone position are shown by LED indicator. The thrust force is not under control but it is only limited by the harp motion. The speed is set preliminary. The decision to stop drilling is taken by the surgeon. The experimental data are obtained for specimen simulating the bi-cortical bone features. They are reported when made under ideal conditions - simulated specimen with constant density (not bone) and flat surface of walls. The stop decision for drilling is manual (not automatic). The surgeon's decision is taken according to the data on the display which may cause a subjective error. The overheating problem prevention is not commented.

- surgical drill device **IntelliSense**

It is developed by "McGinley Orthopedic Innovations", US [16] and has two working regimes: conventional (Free Hand Mode) and bi-cortical. In bi-cortical regime the surgeon receives the signals from the device when the drill bit is close to the end of far cortex. This helps to him to stop drilling on time avoiding undesirable penetration in the soft tissues. The surgeon controls the thrust force himself all the time. No information is given for the criterion to stop rotation after the breakthrough and for penetration of the drill bit after the far cortex end. This system is not a robot according to the accepted definitions but allows receiving information for already drilled depth and far cortex end in real time. Among its disadvantages are no thrust force control, no prevention of overheating, and no automatic detection of breakthrough.

- handheld robotized system **DRIBON** [17].

It is still under development. This system is oriented to bi-cortical drilling only and especially for precise breakthrough detection and automatic stop of drilling. The stop decision is based on control algorithm where error of the feed-back position is analyzed during the motion. Constant speed is set in linear motion law and the maximal thrust force which can be applied is restricted. But the drilling time is over 400 s for cow bone bi-cortical drilling as it is reported standing on the experimental results which is very large time in comparison with the surgical practice. That reflects to high temperature in drilling zone (data for the temperature deviation are not reported) which causes negative results.

## 2. Orthopedic bone drilling robot ODRO

Many papers and books are written which are devoted to various aspects of robots. Lots of authors of different nationalities have given many arguments trying to confirm their arguments concerning the robot understanding, characteristics and definitions [18]. Nevertheless some variations appear about the attempts to formulate a unified definition - the general point of view includes several main features needed to describe a device or machine as a robot. So, these general common characteristics which an object must have to be really called a robot are as follows:

- Mechanical system
- Driving system
- Sensor system
- Computer control system

They are necessary but not sufficient conditions. For example the control system must be considered together with software and corresponding interface which looks after the connection and communication with environment. Moreover, the software must have possibilities for reprogramming the motion of the mechanical system concerning its positioning or trajectory tracking. And the most important thing – the system has to be autonomous one, i.e. it must be able to take decisions of its own. The last characteristic is not fulfilled for the objects operating under human being control. For instance, some people used to call them also as "robots" but that is an error – the true is that they are telemanipulators.

### 2.1 Basic subsystems of the ODRO

ODRO - Orthopedic Drilling Robot [11, 19] consists of control/power block and handheld surgical drill (**Figure 1**).

#### *2.1.1 Mechanical system*

Mechanical structure (surgical drill) with two degrees of freedom is proposed (**Figure 2**). It has one translation and one revolute joint with co-linear axes, where $q_1$ and $q_2$ are corresponding generalized coordinates. The new assembly drawing which corresponds to the new construction is shown in **Figure 3**.

Both actuators are mounted inside the drilling module. All parts of the mechanical module are made by stainless steel material for assuring the sterility requirements. The machine allows gas chemical sterilization before every manipulation.

#### *2.1.2 Driving system*

The drill bit rotation (0–1000 rpm) is realized by BLDC (Brushless Direct Current) motor "MAXON EC-4-pole 30" assuring 1.66 Nm torque (Maxon Motor AG, Shwaiz). These motor types have many advantages. Among them are better speed versus torque characteristics; high dynamic response; high efficiency; long operating life; noiseless operation; higher speed ranges; rugged construction etc. These features make the chosen motor useful for applications especially in cases where the space of work and the motor weight are critical factors.

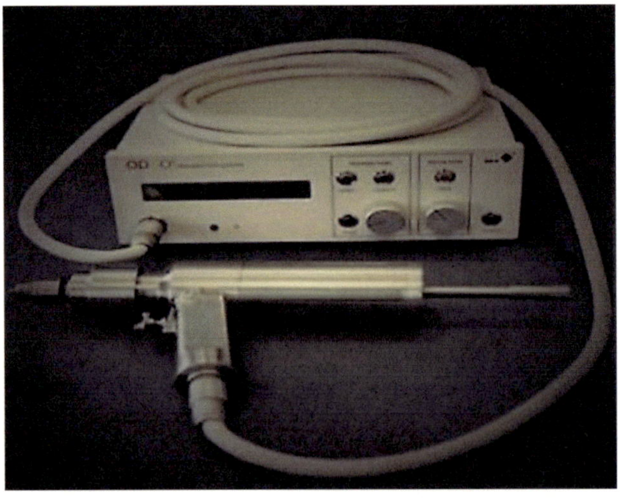

**Figure 1.**
*ODRO – Control block and handheld surgical drill.*

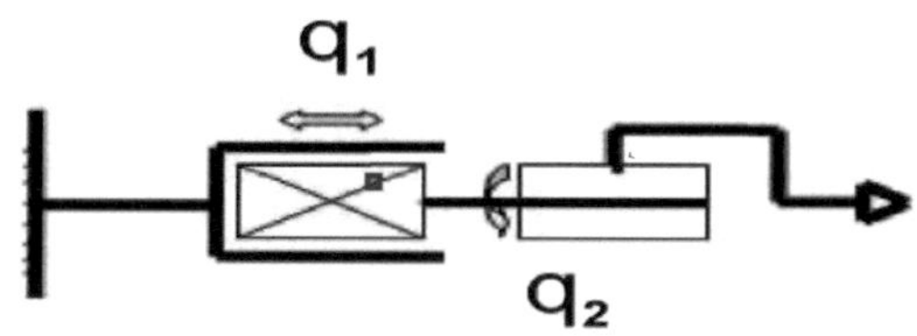


**Figure 2.**
*Kinematic scheme of the mechanical structure.*

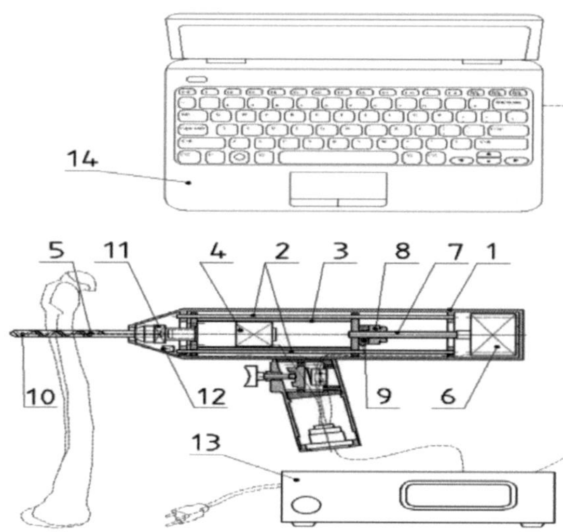


**Figure 3.**
*The new assembly drawing and the numbers related to the main components: BLDC motor MAXON EC-4-pole 30 (number 3); step motor type 43000–17 (number 6) and force sensor LMB-A-200 N (number 8).*

The linear motion (0–100 mm) is driven by step motor type "43000–17" (Haydon Switch & Instrument Inc.) which can apply thrust force up to 120 N in velocity range 0–9 mm/s. It is stepper motor with embedded screw for linear motion. It has high precision at low speeds, small by size and realizes translation of 1 mm for 4032 micro steps.

### *2.1.3 Sensor system*

The system has force feed-back which is assured by force sensor "MLP-25", "Transducer Techniques" having measurement range up to 120 N [19]. In the next version of the system this force sensor is replaced by "LMB-A-200 N (KYOWA)" [11] because it is more compact, lightweight (6 g), has low price and measurement range up to 200 N.

### *2.1.4 Control system*

The control system is on the base of one axis stepper controller/driver TMCM-1110 (TRINAMIC, Hamburg, Germany). This module controls the linear motion and keeps the bone drilling process control program to be realized successfully.

The servo controller/driver "1-Q-CE Amplifier DEC 50-5" with build-in speed PID-regulator controls the BLDC motor.

Terminals for connection with PC are also built-in in the control block. They give a possibility to re-program the software, which is recorded in the "TMCM-1110" module, to change and update the programs and to transfer the information between the control module and PC while the drilling is executed in real time.

## 2.2 Technical data and functional characteristics

### *2.2.1 Technical data of the robotized surgical drill*

- weight – 2.3 kg
- working zone – 0 – 100 mm
- precision – 0.1 mm
- working regime
- "hand"
- automatic
- drill speed (rotation speed) – 0-1000 rpm
- feed rate (translation speed) – 0 – 6 mm/s
- drill (thrust) force – up to 120 N in the feed rate range 0–6 mm/s
- drill torque – 1.66 Nm in the drill speed range 0–1000 rpm
- real time depth measurement of the hole depth
- auto-stop after the end of the far (second) cortex
- minimal drill bit penetration after the end of the far (second) cortex in the range of 0 – 1 mm
- feed rate control during drilling

The following indications can be seen on the control/power block:

- emergency indication
- digital display
- drilling mode buttons
- confirm button

Control systems give information for the drilling execution, for successful end of the task and for emergency situation.

### *2.2.2 Functional characteristics*

Our Orthopedic Drilling Robot has two working modes: manual and automatic. In manual regime it is like a usual drilling device. The rotational speed is regulated by potentiometer in the range 0–1000 rpm.

The automatic working can be separated in three sub-modes:
*Fixed depth* - drilling of a hole with preliminary set depth of the hole in *mm*;
*Cortex I* – first cortex (unicortical) drilling;
*Cortex II* – both cortices (bicortical) drilling.
The latter mode (*Cortex II)* in turn supports three sub-modes:

- Cortex II Full Drill – bicortical drilling and automatic stop after second cortex end registration

- Cortex II Find – drill bit detection the far cortex wall from inside and stop automatically.

- Cortex II Drill – drilling through the near (first) cortex and partially drilling the far (second) one, making a hole with a predetermined depth in [mm].

The working modes are set by the surgeon using four buttons and a potentiometer in combination with a display (**Figures 4–6**). Also it gives information in real time about the duration of the drilling process and about the operation result at the end of the drilling. The drilling is realized with an accuracy of 0.1 mm.

The result is presented on the display after drilling manipulation. The second row of the display screen (**Figure 7**) shows: first number - the thickness of the near cortex (Cortex I); second number - the thickness of the far cortex (Cortex II); third number - the depth of the hole. The second row in **Figure 8** in the same manner shows the thickness of the near cortex (first number), the distance between both cortices (marrow) and the depth of the hole (third number).

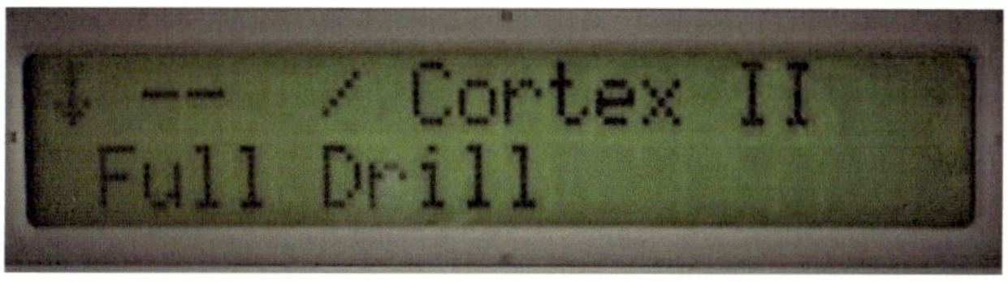


**Figure 4.**
*"Cortex II full drill" mode - bicortical drilling and automatic stop after second cortex end registration.*

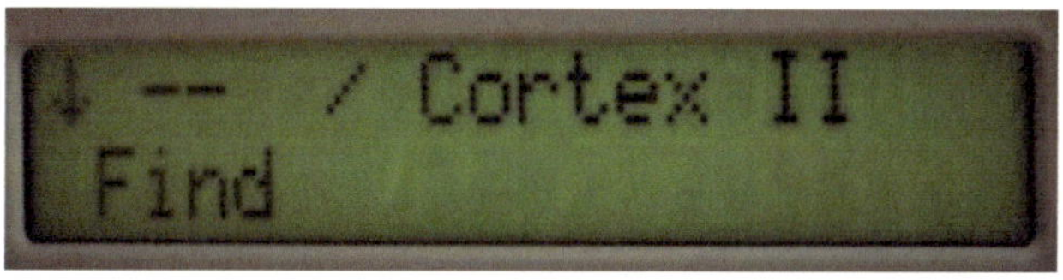


**Figure 5.**
*"Cortex II find" mode - drill bit detection the far cortex wall from inside and stop automatically.*

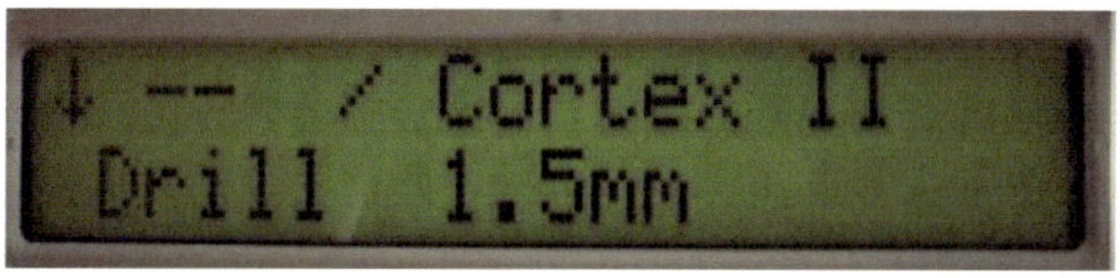


**Figure 6.**
*"Cortex II drill" mode - drilling through the near (first) cortex and partially the far (second) one, making a hole with a 1.5 depth in [mm].*

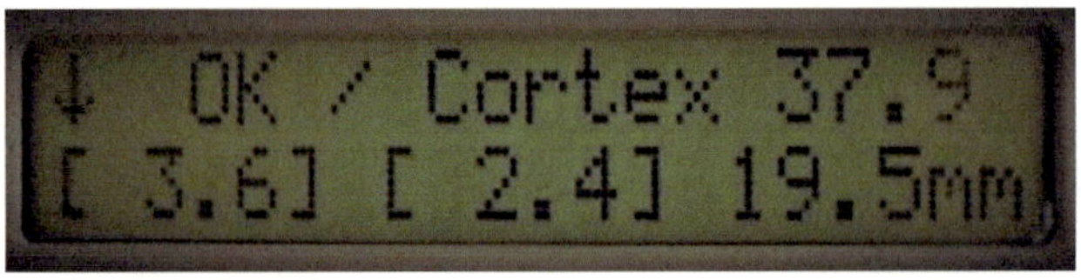


**Figure 7.**
*Information displayed after "Cortex II Full" drill mode.*

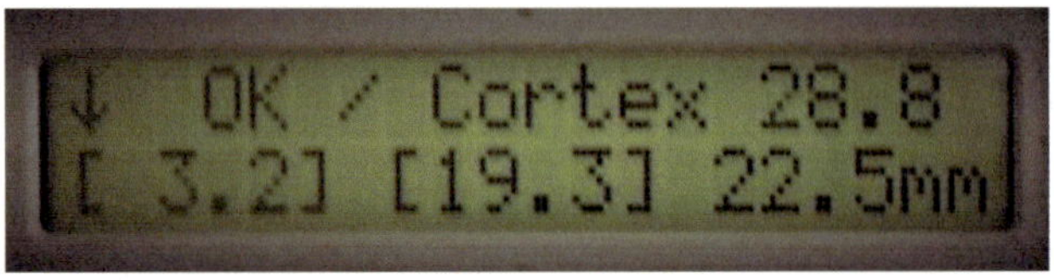


**Figure 8.**
*Information displayed after "Cortex II Find" mode.*

## 3. Bone drilling process execution

The successful realization of drilling manipulation depends on normal functioning of the whole system components – motors, force sensor, controllers, buttons, etc. That means the components have to be tested before the start of manipulation. A procedure 'Self Test' is developed which starts immediately after the power is switched on. The 'Self Test' procedure passes through the following testing steps:

- start button reliability (switch on and switch off)
- ability to find out the initial position (Reference position)
- ability to receive the force sensor data
- check the translation motion of the step motor (going forth and back the working zone, free motion resistance, check for missing steps)
- check the rotational motion

The force sensor test reports the ability of transferring the data for resistant force at free translation motion forth and back as well as an average value for normal motion which confirms a previously defined and known criterion.

The decision whether the component works right or wrong is taken according to criteria downloaded in the program. The 'Self Test' procedure confirms safe working the whole system. When some differences from the criteria incorporated in the software are registered then the message "Self TEST ERR" appears on the display. The robot cannot be used until the corresponding reasons are eliminated. The message confirming the positive result of the procedure is "Self TEST OK" on the display.

The next step is to set the working mode. Additionally another parameter in [mm] ( $B_{max}$ ) is set which is connected with the patient's safety and it is related to each specific patient. The hole depth cannot exceed $B_{max}$. This parameter depends on the specific task, for example - it can be taken from the x-ray image of the bone before operation. During the drilling at every discretization time interval " $k$ " the current position is compared with $B_{max}$ and then the decision for going on or stop the process is taken.

Then the drilling process can begin.

The drilling process (**Figure 9**) is running when the button of the executive module (start button) is pressed and is held continuously by the surgeon. He can stop the manipulation aiming to set a new working regime or to prevent a drilling error. The manipulation execution goes on after the start button is pressed again and is held until the drilling ends automatically and the drill bit returns to its home (reference) position. During the operation the surgeon must keep firm contact with the bone all the time. When performing the drilling process, the selected drilling mode was indicated on the display.

The control algorithms are realized in the specialized program language (Trinamic Motion Control Language – TMCL) specific for the TMCM (Trinamic Motion Control Module) controllers in the program environment TMCL-IDE. The execution of commands start immediately after the input (direct regime) or the program can be downloaded for autonomous execution in the controller (stand-alone regime). The user is also allowed to input different axes and global parameters which enrich the control algorithms results and make its realization easier. The main control program is structured in separate states - State Search for Contact, State Contact Found, State Drilling, State Check for Missing Steps, State not Contact Found, State Ready etc. In Stand-alone regime the program recognizes the current state for every cycle and executes the corresponding algorithm, taking a decision for going to the next state in dependence on preliminary determined criteria.

The translation motion control during the drilling is based on the force feed-back. A modified PI control law (Eq. (1)) is used to calculate the new position, or the "next target position", (number of steps $\Delta s_k$ where $k$ is the time interval discretization), which the linear motor as well as the drill bit, respectively, must reach in a given interval of time $\Delta t$.

$$\Delta s_k = K_P \varepsilon_k + K_I I_k, \tag{1}$$

where:

$\varepsilon_k = F_r - F_{act}^k$ ; $I_k = \Sigma \varepsilon_i$ , $\left[ i = (k-4),,\ldots,,k \right]$;

$K_P$ and $K_I$ - feed-back coefficients of the proportional and the integral component in the control low;

$F_{act}^k$ - actual thrust force (measured);

$F_r$ - reference force which must be maintained following the created algorithm during the drilling process. The value of $F_r$ is calculated for drilling of each specific (individual) bone and depends on features of the patients, for example health status, age, sex, etc.

Considering our specific task the following comments have to be done. The registration of far cortex from inside the bone and the breakthrough detection depends on the evaluation of the bone density in the current drilling zone. Because of that an integral component $I_{ds}$ (Eq. (2)) is formed as a sliding window in the same drilling zone. By this integral component information is obtained for the change of bone density:

$$I_{ds}^k = \Sigma I_i, \left[ i = (k-n),\ldots k \right], \tag{2}$$

In the last expression "$n$" is the dimension of $I_{ds}$ in the sense of sample discretization. Its value is updated after every $n$ sample. Decreasing of $I_{ds}$ shows higher bone density and its increasing – drilling in lower bone density in comparison with the bone density which corresponds to Reference Force $F_r$ .

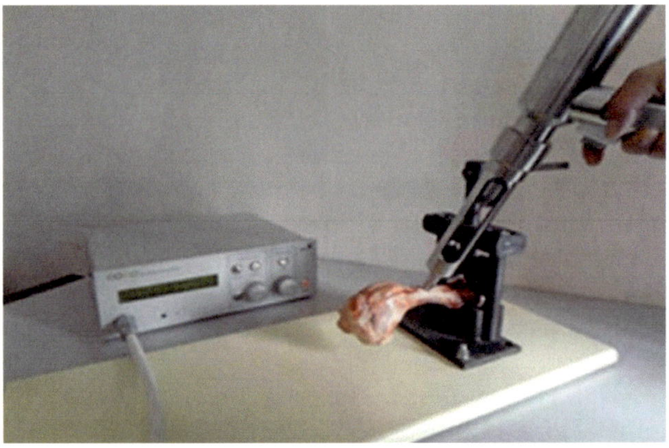

**Figure 9.**
*Bone drilling process.*

The parameter $\Delta I_{ds}$ is formed as a difference between two consecutive values. It gives information for tissue density deviation in current drilling area. The higher the $\Delta I_{ds}$ the bigger is bone density deviation in the current zone in comparison with the zone drilled just before.

Next, the comparison of the value $\Delta I_{ds}$ with some appropriately chosen reference value allows taking a decision for the breakthrough detection of second cortex as well as the far cortex registration. The dimension of $I_{ds}$ from view point of number of subtractions ($\varepsilon_k = F_r - F_{act}^k$) assures the accurate monitoring the tendency of increasing or decreasing the bone density and in the same time minimizes the "not typical force sensor data" in the drilling area.

The dimension of $I_{ds}$ from view point of number of samples of discretization is in connection with the extent of the drill bit penetration when it starts moving in low density area.

Once the drilling process is completed according to the selected operating mode, the result of the operation is presented on the display.

## 4. Areas of application and experimental results

### 4.1 Long bone fractures

The most common fractures are long bone fractures. In the treatment of long bone fractures by osteosynthesis, the most commonly used manipulation is bicortical drilling.

The main problem during bicortical bone drilling is the second cortex breakthrough detection and drill bit penetration value. The average soft tissue penetration in bi-cortical drilling manipulations is 6.31 mm when drilling is executed manually [20]. Furthermore, there is a significant difference in plunging (soft tissue penetration) depth when sharp or blunt drill bit was being used. Surgeons, regardless of their experience level, when used blunt drill bit, penetrate over 20 mm in normal bone and over 10 mm in osteoporotic bone [21]. This means that there is a risk of tendon or blood vessel rupture and protection of the posterior bone wall is required (leading to additional tissue excision).

When performing the drilling by the orthopedic bone drilling robot ODRO, the manipulation can be conditionally described by several stages: searching the contact with the first cortex; its drilling; automatic stop; searching the contact with the second cortex; its drilling; automatic stop; going to reference position after the drilling end.

In **Figures 10** and **11** experimental results are presented for the current position and the feed rate consequently during a bicortical mid-diaphyseal pork femur bone drilling procedure.

**Figures 12** and **13** present experimental data for thrust force variation during bicortical pig femur bone drilling when using a new drill bit (**Figure 12**) and a drill bit after 35 drillings (**Figure 13**).

The time is expressed in arbitrary units (AU) of measurement where 1 unit is defined as the scoring time, i.e. the interval of time between two measurements.

During bicortical bone drilling process the feed rate takes various values in any stage in the range 0.5-6 mm/s. These values depend on drill bit position and real time force sensor data.

The first drilling stage is illustrated in **Figure 11** (search of contact with first cortex). Its parameters are feed rate 6 mm/s and drill speed 0 rpm. When the contact is realized, the feed rate stops (at 145 AU in **Figure 11**) and the drill speed is switched on. As the tubular bones generally have not flat shape the drill bit may slip from the needed point of drilling start. That can be notices and corrected by the surgeon

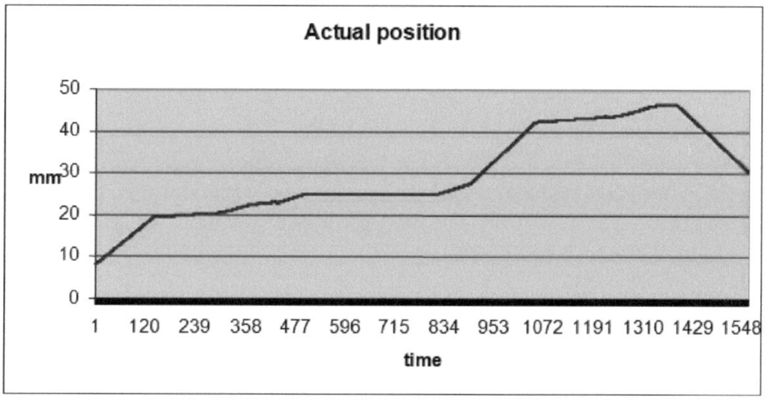


**Figure 10.**
*Actual position [mm] versus time during drilling. Maximal drilling feed rate 2 mm/s; drill bit 2.8 mm; total time 21.016 s, 1561 AU.*

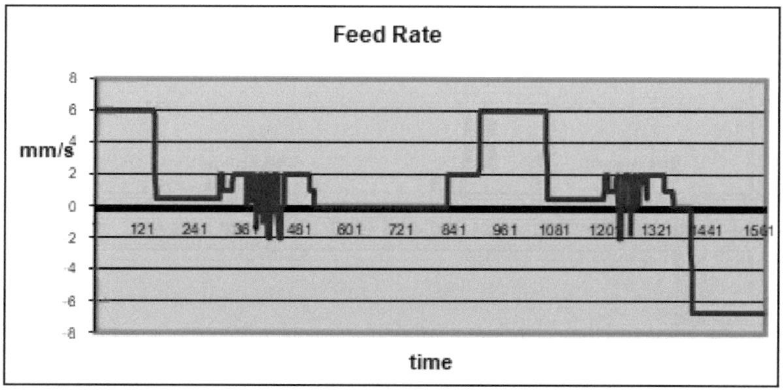


**Figure 11.**
*Feed rate [mm/s] versus time during drilling. Maximal drilling feed rate 2 mm/s; drill bit 2.8 mm; total time 21.016 s, 1561 AU.*

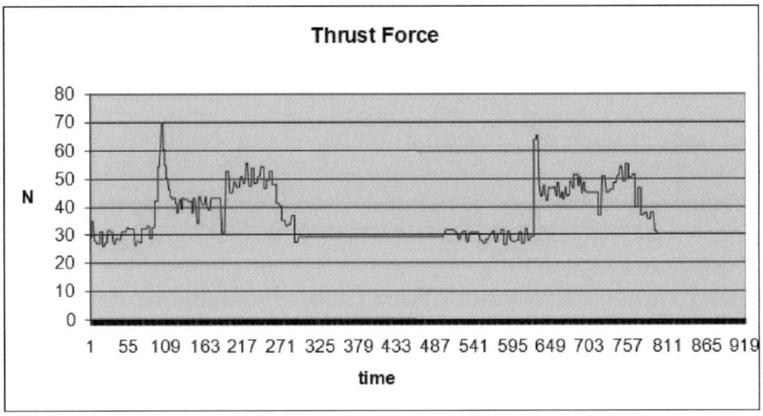


**Figure 12.**
*Thrust force [N] versus time during drilling maximal drilling feed rate 2 mm/s; new drill bit 2.8 mm; total time 18.297 s, 919 AU. Drilling time (101–796 AU) – 13.85 s.*

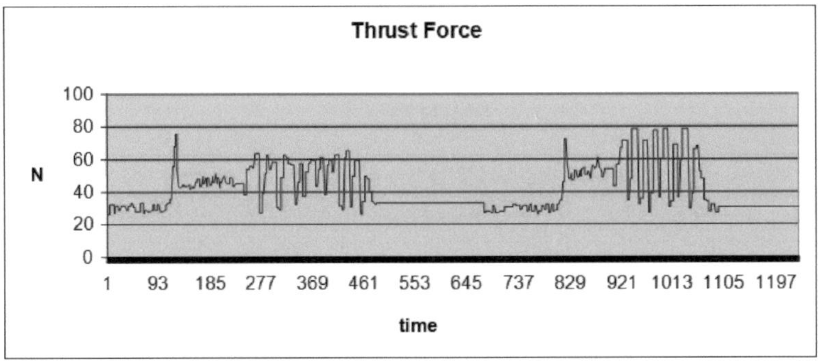


**Figure 13.**
*Thrust force [N] versus time during drilling. Maximal drilling feed rate 2 mm/s; hole-used 35 times drill bit 2.8 mm; total time 24.828 s, 1,239 AU. Drilling time (128–1,097 AU) – 19.42 s.*

in the case of first cortex but for drilling the second cortex such a slippage (which starts from inside the bone) cannot be avoided. It results to drill bit bending which reflects to hole inaccuracy, bigger friction and heat generation [1].

The second drilling stage (drilling start) begins after the contact is established. In order to eliminate the case of drill bit bending at the first cortex entrance site the drilling is executed with a feed rate 0.5 mm/s (from 148 to 288 AU in **Figure 11**). During this time interval the thrust force is identified for the first cortex (thrust force = 40 N, **Figure 12**). So that a thrust forces reference value is set to 50 N (**Figure 12**) for the first cortex wall for further drilling.

At the third drilling stage the feed rate has maximal value 2 mm/s. The fourth drilling stage indicates the end of the first cortex drilling at 509 AU in **Figure 11** and the drilling automatically stops; drill speed and feed rate become equal to 0 (the fifth drilling stage) according to the auto-stop criterion [22].

The registration of the inner (or outer) wall of the near (or far) cortex and the decision to stop the drilling process depends on the bone density evaluation in the current drilling zone (thrust force = 40 N, **Figure 12**) [22]. After pressing the start button again the drilling process starts at 817 AU in **Figure 11**. The drill speed is 1000 rpm and the drill bit movement is executed with feed rate of 2 mm/s (along 2 mm distance - from 818 to 892 AU in **Figure 11**).

The drill bit does not penetrate through the bone wall entirely when the first cortex wall drilling is finished from the "robot viewpoint" (the penetration is less than 1 mm but the stop decision works out successfully). This way, delamination of bone layers at the exit of the drill bit at the second wall of the first cortex is eliminated. Then the process continues with feed rate 6 mm/s until the second cortex contact is reached (in the same style like the first drilling stage but now for the second cortex) – feed rate 6 mm/s (893–1046 AU in **Figure 11**). When the second cortex contact is registered (1047 AU in **Figure 11**) the drilling process continues according to the algorithm steps already described up to now for the first cortex drilling until an automatic stop is realized when the second cortex drilling is finished. Then the drill bit was extracted back to the reference position (after 1400 AU in **Figure 11**) with negative value (6 mm/s) of the feed rate (the fifth drilling stage for the second cortex).

The drilling of the first or second cortex, which is in the interval of 299–509 AU in **Figure 11**, is executed with feed rate not greater than 2 mm/s. This value changes during the drilling process in dependence on the force sensor data.

When the resistant force values become less than the reference force, drilling is executed with feed rate 2 mm/s, for example in the intervals 320–351 AU and 438–497 AU in **Figure 11**. Feed rate values less than 2 mm/s correspond to slower translation motion (the resistant force values are higher than the reference value) and also correspond to application of a smaller thrust force (352–399 AU in **Figure 11**).

Thus, the negative feed rate values correspond to drill bit back-motion while a recurring overshoot of the reference value occurs (for example 400–431 AU in **Figure 11**). That is in agreement with the scientific reports of ultrasonically-assisted drilling method (UAD) [23–27]. This is a concept of minimizing the thrust force during drilling. The original idea of this approach is a module coupled with the drill bit, realizing the micro back translation motions with 5-25 μm amplitude and 10–30 kHz frequency. The advantages of UAD in comparison with conventional drilling reflect in a decrease of force from 60–65 N to 35–38 N (for UAD) [23, 25].

When the drill position becomes close to the second cortex outer surface (which can be recognized by additional criteria) then the feed rate decreases to 1 mm/s (498–508 AU in **Figure 11**). The reduction of the feed rate aims to guarantee a minimal penetration (maximum 1 mm) in the tissue outside the bone. Additionally, reduction the speed to 1 mm/s (respectively the thrust force) at the end of drilling allows forming accurately the breakthrough itself, i.e. without bone debris.

The feed rate control has important role from viewpoint of usage of spoiled drill bits which occurs very often in orthopedic practice. It is confirmed by a report where about 600 and more drillings are executed [28]. The dulled drill bits cause higher temperature in the drilling area. The maximal temperature reached by a bit taken from the operation room is $54.5^{0}$ C [28, 29]. A proportional relationship is observed between the intensity of wear and the temperature increase and the same can be said for cutting forces [29].

After the end of every concrete drilling, the result is shown on the display. In **Figures 14** and **15** results of the drilling in both cases concerning the new and the used drill bits (see **Figures 12** and **13**) are shown on the display. The thickness of the

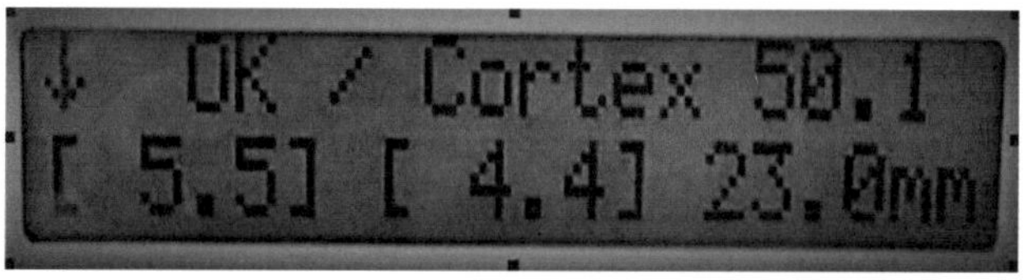


**Figure 14.**
*The result of the drilling process; new drill bit 2.8 mm.*

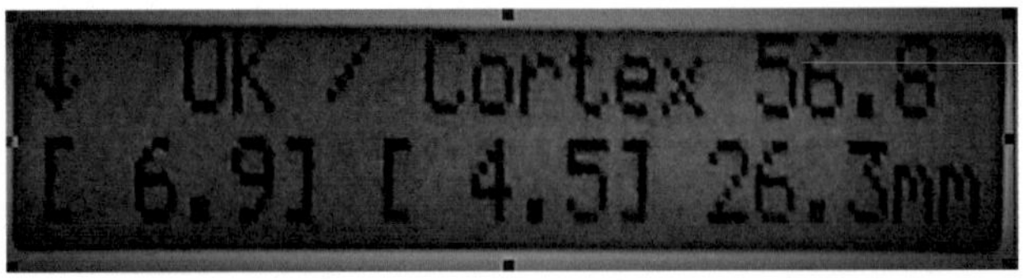


**Figure 15.**
*The result of the drilling process; hole-used 35 times drill bit 2.8 mm.*

near cortex (Cortex I), the thickness of the far cortex (Cortex II) and the depth of the hole are shown in the second row on the display.

At equal drilling conditions – drilling process control algorithm, drill bit diameter, bone specimen, drilling area – the following can be seen in **Figures 12** and **13**: for new drill bit max thrust force is 55 N; for used drill bit max thrust force is 80 N; for new drill bit the hole depth is 23 mm for 13.85 s duration and for used drill bit the hole depth is 26.3 mm for 19.42 s respectively.

At automatic drilling the reasons for the negative final result caused by dulled drill bits should be minimized by feed rate control [30]. Also, it successfully solves the problem of higher drill bit penetration after the end of second cortex. It is realized by feed rate reduction to 1 mm/s just before the breakthrough.

### 4.2 Hip fractures

Generally said a hip-fracture is a break in the upper part of the femur bone. It occurs mostly to the patients over 60 years old. Worldwide the human population growing older is a clear tendency. It is expected such changes can cause higher number of hip fractures increasing from 1.66 million in 1990 to 6.26 million in 2050 [31]. Moreover, it is proved the hip fractures are one of the main reasons for mortality of the old people. For example the mortality to the end of the first year after the trauma reaches 27.3% depending on the kind and the type of hip fracture treatment [32]. These data underline the social importance of the problem and lots of researches concern their efforts for optimization of hip fracture treatment and maximal patient's recovery.

For metal osteosynthesis of proximal femur fracture the implant is placed (inserted) through the lateral cortex and anchors into the hip head. The post-operative complications, which often occur at fracture treatment by osteosynthesis and require an implant change or arthroplasty, are the so called hip head re-fracture and implant penetration into the joint capsule.

The main reason for that is a wrong positioning of the screws into the femoral head–neck fragment. As a criterion for implant position the so called Tip-to-Apex Distance index (TAD – index) is used. The optimal positioning corresponds to TAD – index minimization. For instance, it is the best factor of prognosis to realize the cut out of the hip head and when the TAD – index is less than 24 mm, the cut outs are unfortunately not registered [33]. That means drilling through the lateral cortex along the hip neck axis, which ends when the drill bit tip is as much as possible close to the far cortex of the hip head.

The experimental results for far cortex registration during proximal pig femur drilling along the neck axis are presented in **Figure 16**. The measured proximal femur length is 65 mm. The hip head cortex registration is in a distance 61.7 mm from the contact point [34].

The hip head cortex registration occurs at 1107 AU in **Figure 16** where $I_{ds}$ again takes values less than zero. Then the drilling automatically stops and the robot takes out the drill bit at the initial position.

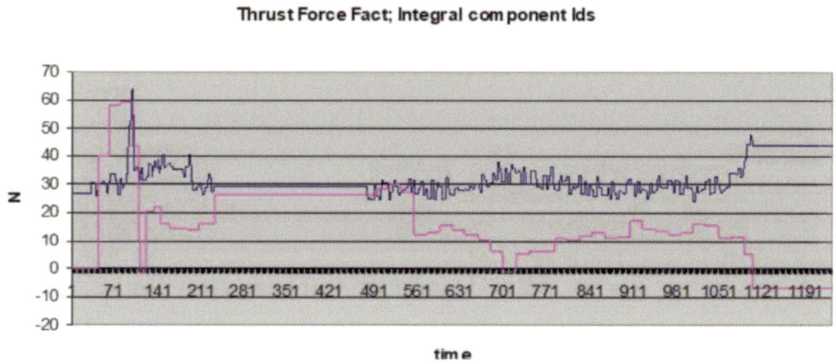


**Figure 16.**
*Far cortex registration during proximal pig femur bone drilling along the neck axis. Maximal drilling feed rate = 4 mm/s; drill bit 2.8 mm; Total time 24.84 s, 1235 AU; hole depth 61.7 mm. The values of the integral component $I_{ds}$ (red line) are scaled by multiplication of $10^{-1}$.*

For some types of fractures, like a midshaft clavicle fractures, it is advisable to fix the implants without drilling the second cortex. Comprising uni-cortical far-cortex–abutting locking screw fixation with bi-cortical fixation, it can be seen that both types of fixation have similar mechanical properties concerning axial and torsional loads in the case when the far cortex penetration not occurs [35]. Uni-cortical far-cortex-abutting locking screw fixation risks far cortex penetration which requires protection of near anatomical structures [35]. Drilling modes of ODRO as Cortex I (unicortical drilling), Cortex II Find and Cortex II Drill can be used in such cases.

One more application of ODRO is related to the proximal humerus fractures. This problem is discussed in [36–38] and here we will present it briefly by citing some sentences from there aiming to show this problem clearer way.

Proximal humerus fractures may occur at the surgical neck, anatomic neck, greater tuberosity, and lesser tuberosity. They are common fractures which can often be seen in elder patients with osteoporotic bone after low level energy impacts. These patients usually have very low bone mineral density and that makes fracture fixation much complicated. Proximal humerus fractures account for 5% of all fractures and represent the third most common osteoporotic fracture [36]. The incidence of these injuries is expected to increase due to the aging population and the growing prevalence of osteoporosis [37].

Within the surgically treated fractures open reduction and internal fixation using locked plates is the most commonly applied joint-preserving treatment of proximal humerus fractures [38]. Failure rates of locked plating depend on the so-called "overdrilling". Perforation of the joint surface during pilot hole drilling is referred to as "overdrilling" [37]. Possible reasons for the overdrilling include: the restricted tactile feedback especially in osteoporotic bone; the spherical morphology of the humeral head that, together with the angulated locking screw projections, make interpreting of intra-operative X-ray images very complicated; the surgeons' experience level; the blunt drill bit [37].

Precision drilling to the correct depth could help prevention of overdrilling and significantly increases endurance until screw perforation failure, i.e. reduce failure rates of locked plating in an unstable proximal humerus fractures [37].

The drilling mode "Fixed depth" of ODRO (preliminary set depth of the hole in mm) can be used in such cases when ODRO is applied. When working in this mode, the set depth of the hole is realized with an accuracy of 0.1 mm.

During bicortical drilling, when the drilling is done manually, the magnitude of the drill bit penetration requires protection of the posterior bone wall. That means the obligatory cutting of the tissues immediately after it.

The drilling through the lateral cortex along the hip neck axis in fractures of the hip joint, as close as possible to the distal hip head cortex, can be performed successfully manually only under continuous X-ray control. This is of the utmost importance for stable fixation of the implant. The use of ODRO in this type of manipulations allows the use of surgical techniques associated with minimally invasive surgery.

## 5. Discussion and conclusion

The process of bone drilling is characterized by a set of input and output parameters. The input parameters define the conditions under which the process takes place, while the output parameters determine the outcome of the process.

Many scientific investigations are done concerning input parameters as drill speed, feed rate, different types of drill bit, its diameter, bone type and drilling methods. These parameters are responsible for heat generation, micro cracks, hole delamination, breakthrough detection and penetration. The results are reported only for the case when one of the parameters has a fixed value (drill speed) and the other one has a discrete variation (feed rate) or vise versa.

The experiments are made by Computer Numerical Control (CNC) machines or CNC milling machines [39–41]. The purpose is to find such combinations of input parameters which may guarantee optimal output parameters during the process of bone drilling.

The difference between the experimental results of various studies arise for the sake of the wide variety of test conditions used by researchers regarding drill-bit diameter, drill bit type, rotational speed, feed rate and bone type. [42]. However, the following dependencies stand out:

Increasing the feed rate leads to:

- reducing the drilling time, i.e. reducing heat generation [43, 44], i.e. reduces the risk of thermal osteonecrosis
- increase of the thrust force [42], i.e. increase the risk of bone damage (traumatic osteonecrosis)
- Increasing the drill speed leads to:
- increase in temperature [43, 45, 46], i.e. the risk of thermal osteonecrosis
- decrease of thrust force [42], i.e. reduces the risk of bone damage (traumatic osteonecrosis)

Summarizing, to minimize heat generation during drilling (avoid thermal osteonecrosis) one should work with the highest possible value of feed rate and the lowest possible value of drill speed. To avoid traumatic osteonecrosis it is necessary to work with the lowest possible value of feed rate and with the highest possible value of drill speed.

Therefore, there are conflicting requirements regarding the values of the parameters drill speed and feed rate, which should be maintained (implemented) during the bone drilling process in order to obtain an optimal result.

During the manual drilling these parameters are controlled by the surgeon on the base of his practical skills. But the optimal results of the manipulations can be assured only when the input parameters are under control during the automatic execution of the drilling process. This is the main reason for the appearance of the handheld robotized systems.

As it was said, the purpose of handheld robotized systems development is to reach the accuracy and precise working of the stationary multifunctional robots. In addition, these systems combine robotic drilling technology with the familiarity of traditional, handheld medical drills. Among the important characteristics of the handheld robotized systems must be underlined no requirements of pre-operative planning, calibration, intraoperative navigation systems. Moreover, they are cheaper, easy and convenient for working and maintenance which allows their mass application in surgery practice.

ODRO has some advantages in comparison to other considered systems: an algorithm for synthesis of the referenced feed rate during drilling, ability for far cortex detection from inside the bone, various specialized working regimes. Up to now, according to the author's knowledge, there are no reports for automatic bone drilling handheld systems that do not use a fixed feed rate during the whole drilling process. The only two systems available in the market which are used in hospitals - SMARTdrillR and IntelliSense orthopedic surgical drill device, also work in fixed feed rate mode. It is important to underline again that the other systems ability of work report only for bicortical drilling. The ODRO system has not only such ability but many additional drilling working modes which were already discussed.

## Acknowledgements

This research is supported by the National Scientific Program eHealth in Bulgaria.

## Conflict of interest

The authors declare no conflict of interest.

## Author details

Tony Boiadjiev[1], George Boiadjiev[2]*, Kamen Delchev[2,3], Ivan Chavdarov[2] and Roumen Kastelov[4]

1 Institute of Information and Communication Technologies, Bulgarian Academy of Sciences, Sofia, Bulgaria

2 Faculty of Mathematics and Informatics, Sofia University, Sofia, Bulgaria

3 Institute of Mechanics, Bulgarian Academy of Sciences, Sofia, Bulgaria

4 Orthopedic and Trauma Clinical Centre, Ministry of Interior, Sofia, Bulgaria

*Address all correspondence to: george@fmi.uni-sofia.bg

## References

[1] Jamil M, Rafique S, Khan AM, Hegab H, Mia M, Gupta MK, Song Q. Comprehensive analysis on orthopedic drilling: A state-of-the-art review. Proc IMechE Part H: J Engineering in Medicine. 2020;234:537-561. DOI: 10.1177/0954411920911283

[2] Augustin G, Zigman T, Davila S, Udilljak T, Staroveski T, Brezak D, et al. Cortical bone drilling and thermal osteonecrosis. Clin Biomech Elsevier. 2012; 27(4): 313-325. DOI: 10.1016/j.clinbiomech.2011.10.010

[3] Torun Y, Pazarcı Ö, Öztürk A. Current Approaches to Bone-Drilling Procedures with Orthopedic Drills. Cyprus J Med Sci. 2020;5(1):93-98. DOI: 10.5152/cjms.2020.1242

[4] Bolland MJ, Hood G, Bastin ST, King AR, Grey A. Bilateral femoral head osteonecrosis after septic shock and multiorgan failure. J. Bone Miner. Res. 2004;19(3):517-520. DOI: 10.1359/JBMR.0301250

[5] Beasley RA. Medical Robots: Current System and Research Directions. Journal of Robotics. 2012;2012:1-14, DOI: 10.1155/2012/401613

[6] Yu F, Li L, Teng H, Shi D, Jiang Q. Robots in orthopedic surgery. Annals of Joint. 2018;3(3):15-21. DOI: 10.21037/aoj.2018.02.01

[7] Hoeckelmann M, Rudas IJ, Fiorini P, Kirchner F, Haidegger T. Current Capabilities and Development Potential in Surgical Robotics. Advanced Robotic Systems. 2015;12(5):61-100. DOI: 10.5772/60133

[8] Davies B, A review of robotics in surgery. Proc IMechE Part H: J Engineering in Medicine. 2000; 214(1): 129-140. DOI: 10.1243/09544110 01535309

[9] Gomes P. Surgical robotics: Reviewing the past, analysing the present, imagining the future. Robotics and Computer-Integrating Manufacturing. 2011;27(2):261-266, DOI:10.1016/j.rcim.2010.06.009.

[10] Sugano N. Computer-assisted orthopedic surgery. Journal of Orthopedic Science. 2003;8(3):442-448. DOI: 10.1007/s10776-002-0623-6

[11] Boiadjiev G, Boiadjiev T, Delchev K, Kastelov R, Chavdarov I, Basic Characteristics of Handheld Robotized Systems in Orthopedic Surgery. 2020 In: Proceedings of the International Conference on Software, Telecommunications and Computer Networks (SoftCOM); 17-19 Sept. 2020; Split, Hvar, Croatia; 2020. p. 1-5, DOI: 10.23919/SoftCOM50211.2020.9238339

[12] ISO 373:2012(en) Robots and robotic devices. Available from: https://www.iso.org/obp/ui/#iso:std:iso:8373:ed-2:v1:en

[13] Herron DM, Marohn M, SAGES–MIRA Robotic Surgery Consensus Group. A consensus document on robotic surgery. Surgical Endoscopy. 2008;22(2):313-325. DOI: 10.1007/s00464-007-9727-5

[14] SMARTdrill 6.0. Available from: https://smartmeddevices.com/smartdrill-6-0/#

[15] SMARTdrill 6.0 Now Available for Orthopedic Surgery. Available from: https://www.prnewswire.com/news-releases/smartdrill-6-0-now-available-for-orthopedic-surgery-300809777.html

[16] IntelliSense Drill Technology. Available from: https://www.mcginleyorthopedicinnovations.com/

[17] Louredo M, Diaz I, Gil J. DRIBON: A mechatronic bone

drilling tool. Mechatronics. 2012;22(8):1060-1066. DOI: 10.1016/j.mechatronics.2012.09.001

[18] Nakano E. Introduction to robotics. Moscow: Mir; 1988. 334 p. ISBN 4-274-08531-7. (in Russian)

[19] Boiadjiev G, Kastelov R, Boiadjiev T, Kotev V, Delchev K, Zagurski K, Vitkov V. Design and performance study of an orthopaedic surgery robotized module for automatic bone drilling. J Medical Robotics and Computer Assisted Surgery. 2013;9(4):455-463. DOI:10.1002/rcs.1479

[20] Clement H, Heidari N, Grechenig W, Weinberg AM, Pichler W. Drilling, not a benign procedure: Laboratory simulation of true drilling depth. Journ. Injury. 2012;43(6):950-952. DOI: 10.1016/j.injury.2011.11.017

[21] Alajmo G, Schlegel U, Gueorguiev B, Matthys R, Gautier E. Plunging when Drilling: Effect of Usiing Blunt Drill Bits. J Orthop Trauma. 2012;26(8):482-467. DOI: 10.1097/BOT.0b013e3182336ec3

[22] Boiadjiev T, Kastelov R, Boiadjiev G, Delchev K, Zagurski K. Automatic Bone Drilling by Femoral Head Structure Detection. Biotechnology & Biotechnological Equipment. 2018;32(3):785-794. DOI: 10.1080/13102818.2017.1407256

[23] Alam K, Mitrofanov AV, Silberschmidt VV. Experimental investigations of forces and torque in conventional and ultrasonically-assisted drilling of cortical bone. Medical Engineering & Physics. 2011;33:234-239. DOI: 10.1016/j.medengphy.2010.10.003

[24] Alam K, Hassan E, Bahadur I. Experimental measurements of temperatures in ultrasonically assisted drilling of cortical bone. Biotechnology & Biotechnological Equipment. 2015;29(4):753-757. DOI: 10.1080/13102818.2015.1034176

[25] Singh RP, Pandey PM, Mridha, AR, Joshi T. Experimental investigations and statistical modeling of cutting force and torque in rotary ultrasonic bone drilling of human cadaver bone. Proc IMechE Part H: J Engineering in Medicine. 2020;234(2):148-162. DOI: 10.1177/0954411919889913

[26] Gupta V, Pandey PM, Gupta RK, Mridha AR. Rotary ultrasonic drilling on bone: A novel technique to put an end to thermal injury to bone. Proc IMechE Part H: Journal of Engineering in Medicine. 2017;231(3):189-196. DOI: 10.1177/0954411916688500

[27] Shakouri E, Sadeghi MH, Karafi MR, Maerefat M, Farzin M. An in vitro study of thermal necrosis in ultrasonic-assisted drilling of bone. Proc IMechE Part H: Journal of Engineering in Medicine. 2015;229(2):137-149. DOI: 10.1177/0954411915573064

[28] Bertollo N, Walsh WR. Drilling of Bone: Practicality, Limitations and Complications Associated with Surgical Drill-Bits. In: Klika V editor. Biomechanics in Applications, London: IntechOpen; 2011. p. 53-83. DOI: 10.5772/20931

[29] Staroveski T, Brezak D, Udiljak T. Drill wear monitoring in cortical bone drilling. Medical Engineering and Physics. 2015;37(6):560-566. DOI: 10.1016/j.medengphy.2015.03.014

[30] Boiadjiev T, Boiadjiev G, Delchev K, Chavdarov I, Kastelov R. Feed rate control in robotic bone drilling process. Proc IMechE Part H: Journal of Engineering in Medicine. 2020: 1-8. DOI: 10.1177/0954411920975890

[31] Dennison E, Mohamed MA, Cooper C. Epidemiology of osteoporosis. Rheum Dis Clin North Am. 2006;32(4): 617-29. DOI: 10.1016/j.rdc.2006.08.003

[32] Panula J, Pihlajamäki H, Mattila VM, Jaatinen P, Vahlberg T, P. Aarnio, Kivelä SL. Mortality and cause of death in hip fracture patients aged 65 or older - a population-based study. BMC Musculoskelet Disord. 2011;12:105. DOI: 10.1186/1471-2474-12-105

[33] Baumgaertner MR, Curtin SL, Lindskog DM, Keggi JM. The value of the tip-apex distance in predicting failure of fixation of peritrochanteric fractures of the hip. J Bone Joint Surg [Am]. 1995;77:1058-1064. DOI: 10.2106/00004623-199507000-00012

[34] Boiadjiev, Boiadjiev G, Delchev K, Chavdarov I, Kastelov R, Automatic bone drilling in hip fractures osteosynthesis. Journal of Theoretical and Applied Mechanics. 2019;49(1):94-104. DOI: 10.7546/JTAM.49.19.01.09

[35] Croley JS, Morris R, Amin A, Lindsey R, Gugala Z. Biomechanical Comparison of Bicortical, Unicortical, and Unicortical Far-Cortex-Abutting Screw Fixations in Plated Comminuted Midshaft Clavicle Fractures. The Journal of Hand Surgery. 2016;41(6):703-710. DOI: 10.1016/j.jhsa.2016.04.001

[36] Court-Brown CM, Caesar B. Epidemiology of adult fractures: a review. Injury. 2006;37:691-697. DOI: 10.1016/j.injury.2006.04.130

[37] Burkhard B, Schopper C, Ciric D, Mischler D, Gueorguiev B, Varga P. Overdrilling increases the risk of screw perforation in locked plating of complex proximal humeral fractures – A biomechanical cadaveric study. Journal of Biomechanics, 2021;117. DOI: 10.1016/j.jbiomech.2021.110268.

[38] Launonen AP, Lepola V, Saranko A, Flinkkila T, Laitinen M, Mattila VM. Epidemiology of proximal humerus fractures. Arch. Osteoporos. 2015;10:209-2013. DOI: 10.1007/s11657-015-0209-4

[39] Wang W, Shi Y, Yang N, Yuan X. Experimental analysis of drilling process in cortical bone. Medical Engineering & Physics. 2014;36:261-266. DOI: 10.1016/j.medengphy.2013.08.006

[40] Pandey RK, Panda SS. Evaluation of delamination in drilling of bone. Medical Engineering and Physics. 2015:37 (7):657-664. DOI: 10.1016/j.medengphy.2015.04.008

[41] Karaca F, Aksakal B. Effects of various drilling parameters on bone during implantology: An in vitro experimental study. Acta of Bioengineering and Biomechanics. 2013;15(4):25-32. DOI: 10.5277/abb130404

[42] Lughmani W, Bouazza-Marouf K, Ashcroft I. Drilling in cortical bone: A Finite element model and experimental investigations. Journal of the Mechanical Behavior of Biomedical Materials.2015;42:32-42. DOI: 10.1016/j.jmbbm.2014.10.017

[43] Augustin G, Davila S, Mihoci K, Udiljak T, Vedrina D, Antabak A. Thermal osteonecrosis and bone drilling parameters revisited. Arch Orthop Trauma Surg. 2008;128:71-77. DOI: 10.1007/s00402-007-0427-3

[44] Chen Y, Hsiao C, Ciou J, Tsai Y, Tu Y. Effects of implant drilling parameters for pilot and twist drills on temperature rise in bone analog and alveolar bones. Medical Engineering and Physics. 2016;38:1314-1321. DOI: 10.1016/j.medengphy.2016.08.009

[45] Fernandes M, Fonseca E, Jorge R, Manzanares M, Dias M. Effect of drill speed on the strain distribution during drilling of bovine and human bones. Journal of Mechanical Engineering and

Biomechanics. 2018;2(5):69-74. DOI: 10.24243/JMEB/2.5.170

[46] Hou Y, Li C, Ma H, Zhang Y, Yang M, Zhang X. An Experimental Research on Bone Drilling Temperature in Orthopaedic Surgery. The Open Materials Science Journal. 2015;9:178-188. DOI: 10.2174/1874088X01509010178